WHO'S AFRAID OF BUTTERFLIES?

Also by Dr Stephen Juan

Only Human: Why We React, How We Behave, What We Feel

All Too Human

A Study Shows: What's New in Child Health & Development
for Parents & Professionals

A Study Shows II: More of What's New in Child Health & Development
for Parents & Professionals

Parenting, Child Development and Child Health (Volume 1)

Parenting, Child Development and Child Health (Volume 2)

The Odd Body: Mysteries of Our Weird and Wonderful Bodies Explained

The Odd Body 2: More Mysteries of Our Weird and Wonderful
Bodies Explained

The Odd Body 3: Still More Mysteries of Our Weird and Wonderful
Bodies Explained

The Odd Brain: Mysteries of Our Weird and Wonderful Brains Explained

The Odd Sex: Mysteries of Our Weird and Wonderful Sex Lives Explained

Can Kissing Make You Live Longer? Body and Behaviour Mysteries Explained

WHO'S AFRAID OF BUTTERFLIES?

Our FEARS and PHOBIAS NAMED and EXPLAINED

Dr Stephen Juan

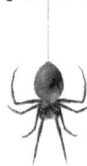

HarperCollins*Publishers*

HarperCollins*Publishers*

First published in Australia in 2011
by HarperCollins*Publishers* Australia Pty Limited
ABN 36 009 913 517
harpercollins.com.au

Copyright © Dr Stephen Juan 2011

The right of Dr Stephen Juan to be identified as the author of this
work has been asserted by him under the *Copyright Amendment
(Moral Rights) Act 2000*.

HarperCollins*Publishers*
25 Ryde Road, Pymble, Sydney NSW 2073, Australia
31 View Road, Glenfield, Auckland 0627, New Zealand
A 53, Sector 57, Noida, UP, India
77–85 Fulham Palace Road, London W6 8JB, United Kingdom
2 Bloor Street East, 20th floor, Toronto, Ontario M4W 1A8, Canada
10 East 53rd Street, New York NY 10022, USA

National Library of Australia Cataloguing-in-Publication entry:

Juan, Stephen.
    Who's afraid of butterflies? : our fears and phobias named
    and explained / Stephen Juan.
    ISBN: 978 0 7322 9051 1 (pbk.)
    Includes bibliographical references.
    Phobias. Fear. Emotions.
616.85225

Cover design: Design by Committee
Original internal design by Alicia Freile, Tango Media, adapted by HarperCollins Design Studio
Typeset in Dante MT 11/16pt by Kirby Jones

To all of us — in the hope that we each may face and overcome
our phobias and fears with understanding and courage

Contents

Chapter 1
Introduction

"Fear is a great weapon of the state.
When a people fear they obey.
Like children, when promised protection they follow."
Adolf Hitler (1889–1945)

"There would be no one to frighten you if you refused to
be afraid."
Mohandas K. Gandhi (1896–1948)

Humans are driven by fear. It seems that at no other time in our history have we had so many fears and allowed them to determine so much of what we do. We fear for our safety (crime and terrorism), our economy (the high cost of living, unemployment, interest rates, the excesses of the banking sector, the greed of big business), our environment (water shortages, energy needs, global warming), our fellow humans (population pressures, religious fundamentalism) and even our own selves. Our leaders know that we are driven by fear and, like many in the advertising industry, cynically use this fact to manipulate and control us. We give up our cherished freedoms for the security of a police state (CCTVs on public streets, full-body scanning at airports, secret surveillance of phone calls and emails, privacy and civil liberties violations of many kinds) because of our fears. After the 9/11 attack in the US, some of us would even believe in violations of the laws of physics if told it's for our protection — all due to fears.

1

This book is about phobias (irrational fears). Phobias exist at the outer reaches of the continuum of our fears. Anything can be the source of a phobia. The phobias discussed in Chapters 2 through 19 and listed in Chapter 24 show just how diverse the sources of extreme fears can be. Reading this list alone will fascinate and shock you. It may make you laugh, feel disgusted or cause you to ask: "Can someone really be afraid of *that?*" But rest assured. All of the phobias in this book are genuine. Someone, somewhere, suffers from it — perhaps even your boss, your newsagent or your next-door neighbour.

WHAT IS A PHOBIA?

A phobia is an anxiety disorder that consists of an extreme, excessive and unreasonable fear and the behaviours associated with that fear. "Phobia" is from the Greek word *phobos* meaning "fear, horror or aversion". In a phobia, the fear results from the exposure to the presence, or merely the anticipation of the exposure to the presence, of a specific object or situation. This object or situation is called the phobic stimulus. The behaviour produced by the phobia, in the form of anxiety and panic, is called a phobic response. The person who suffers from a phobia is called a phobic, or a phobe when used as a suffix (as in Claustrophobe — someone who is irrationally fearful of enclosed spaces). The phobic has a compelling desire to avoid the phobic stimulus in order to avoid the phobic response. If the phobic stimulus is not avoided then the phobic response interferes with normal behaviours. This is why a phobia is a problem for the phobic: phobias get in the way of normal living.[1]

There is often a fine line between a fear and a phobia. A fear is rational while a phobia is irrational. A phobia *must* interfere with common everyday personal functioning of common everyday life. For example, if you are afraid of being a passenger in a car (Motorphobia), then your ability to travel in modern society is seriously restricted.

However, if you are afraid of being a passenger in a car when someone drunk is at the wheel, that is not a phobia; indeed, it is good sense.

If you are afraid of falling off Mt Everest, you do not have Acrophobia (irrational fear of high places, including fear of mountains). Few of us attempt to climb Mt Everest and climbing Mt Everest is certainly not a normal occurrence in daily life. But even here there may be a fine line between fear and phobia: if you could not bear even to look at a picture of Mt Everest for fear of falling off it, then you may have Acrophobia. Or if you could not face being on, thinking of or travelling to any mountain and not just Mt Everest (the highest mountain in the world), you may have Acrophobia. Finally, if you would not visit a friend who lived in a tall building or someone who lived at the top of a hill because it reminds you of Mt Everest, then you may have Acrophobia.

The test of a phobia is that there must be avoidance that interferes with normal life. In all such cases of determining whether a phobia is truly a phobia, a clinical judgement is required by a professional in psychological health.

CAN ANYTHING BE A PHOBIC STIMULUS?

Almost anything can be a phobic stimulus and provoke a phobic response. The length of the list of phobias in this book will no doubt surprise many readers. Ironically, there is a kind of "democracy" in determining phobias. If something is always or often feared by others as well as you, chances are it is less likely to be a phobia. If something is never or rarely feared by others but is feared by you, chances are it is a phobia. Someone's routine object is someone else's phobia. Take for instance the irrational fear of spiders (Arachnophobia). Some see a spider in their house and remove it; others are petrified even of pictures of spiders. The general rule with phobias is that if something exists, chances are someone, somewhere, will be terrified of it.

The frequency of people suffering from at least one phobia in the population is debatable. As one Harvard Medical School study found, the range of incidence rate is between about 4.3 per cent and 100 per cent of the adult population in industrial nations. However, this study and many like it are based upon self-report. Thus, a more accurate statement from the study is that at least 4.3 per cent of the population *admits* to suffering from a phobia. The same study found that having phobias is the most common mental illness in women and the second-most common mental illness in men above the age of 25. According to Dr Adam Guastella, a senior research fellow in clinical psychology at the University of New South Wales, about 10 per cent of the population suffers a phobia at some stage of their lives. He observes that "[t]he three most common are spiders, heights and snakes. Then other fairly common phobias are things like storms, water, birds, animals such as dogs and cats, those sorts of things."[2]

There are dramatic variations in the rates of phobias between nations and cultures. For example, a Canadian study revealed that while 8.8 per cent of the US population was found to suffer from "specific phobias", only 0.2 per cent of the Northern Ireland population did so by comparison.[3] A recent Australian study found that 2.3 per cent of the country's population suffered from "social phobia".[4] Agoraphobia (fear of public places) is far more common in Australia, New Zealand, Canada, the UK, Europe and the US than it is in Japan.[5] Yet in Japan, a common phobia is *taijin kyofusho*, which is almost nonexistent in the Western world. This is an incapacitating fear of offending or harming others through the perceived or imagined awkwardness of one's own physical defects or behaviour.[6] As distinct as phobias are in the West, in Japan the focus of cognition for a sufferer of this phobia is on the harm to others and not on embarrassment to the self, as in Sociophobia in the West. *Taijin kyofusho* is described by Japanese psychiatrists as a pathological exaggeration of the modesty and sensitive regard for others that is considered proper in normal human interactions in Japan.[7]

HOW DO PHOBIAS DEVELOP?

Ideas about the origins of phobias have probably existed since the beginnings of human thought. In the early 20th century, Sigmund Freud and his colleagues of the psychoanalytic theoretical tradition speculated that young children develop Agoraphobia from fear of helplessness and abandonment by a cold, non-nurturing or abusive mother. The fear is then generalised to a phobia of helplessness or abandonment when out of the safety and security of home. By contrast, adherents of the social-learning school of thought suggest that Agoraphobia may develop because people avoid situations where they have had previous painful or embarrassing experiences. In addition, failed coping strategies and low self-esteem contribute to this.[8–10]

Research indicates that people seem predisposed to develop phobias towards creatures and things that arouse disgust, such as rats (Rodentophobia), spiders (Arachnophobia), blood (Haematophobia) and vomit (Emetophobia).[11] A famous experiment by psychologist Martin Seligman[12] involving electric shocks administered to subjects found, perhaps not surprisingly, that it took fewer shocks to establish a phobia of snakes than a phobia of flowers.[13] A phobia of snakes (Ophidiophobia) is far more common than a phobia of flowers (Anthophobia). Nevertheless, most Anthophobes have no doubt developed their phobia without the help of electric shocks.

Interestingly, research shows that almost half of all people with phobias have never had a painful experience with that particular phobic stimulus.[14] This may indicate that phobics have a considerable ability to project themselves into a phobic stimulus situation or that phobics are quite skilled at avoiding the phobic stimulus, whatever and wherever it may be.

If we hear that someone has, for example, been bitten by a poisonous snake, it is possible for us to become Ophidiophobic towards all snakes. Yet, although almost everyone has witnessed or experienced a car accident in which someone was injured or killed, only a minority of us is phobic of cars (Autokinetophobia), driving a car (Mobilophobia) or being a passenger in a car (Motorphobia).

Perhaps humans are "prepared" to learn certain phobias? Over the three million years of human evolution, people who quickly learned to avoid snakes and other such potential "dangers" probably had a better chance of survival than those who did not, thus transmitting their genes forward. However, taking this logic to extremes, the genes of the biggest coward would become the dominant genes of the species. This embarrassing prospect would seem to be counter-intuitive. It also begs the question, unable as it is to account for a fear of cars where time and exposure have been insufficient to affect evolution. Perhaps evolution favours a middle course? This is somewhere between the extremely fearful (i.e. the phobic) and the extremely non-fearful (i.e. the reckless). Holding reasonable fears is that middle ground of relative safety for ourselves and relatively high probability for our genes to survive into the next generation.

Another possible explanation is that people develop phobias for objects and situations they cannot predict or control. Danger is more stressful when it takes you by surprise. Fear of lightning (Keraunophobia) and fear of thunder (Brontophobia) occur because lightning and thunder are unpredictable and uncontrollable. By contrast, electrical outlets will not take you by surprise. So it is unlikely you or anyone else will develop "electric outlet phobia" specifically, but perhaps there is someone, somewhere, who has. Electrophobia refers to the morbid fear of electricity generally.

Modern neuroscience is revealing that biological factors, such as greater blood flow and metabolism in the right hemisphere than in the left hemisphere of the brain, may also be involved in phobias. Identical twins reared apart sometimes develop the same phobias. One twin became Claustrophobic independently of their twin, according to one study. But it is difficult to know what to make of this.[15]

* * *

DO RECENT DEVELOPMENTS IN NEUROSCIENCE PROVIDE INSIGHTS INTO PHOBIAS AND WHY WE DEVELOP THEM?

Modern neuroscience is revolutionising how we conceive the brain. Thirty years ago we used to hear (and medical schools taught) that the brain stopped changing after it stopped growing at about the age of 20. Instead, the only brain change we could look forward to was the death of brain cells (neurons) beginning at a slow rate in our 20s and happening at an increasing rate as we got older. If we were lucky enough to live to a ripe old age, there was little left of the brain. Our eventual grim fate was dementia and senility. This "fixed" brain idea dominated Western medical science for four centuries. However, based upon advanced technology such as functional magnetic resonance imaging (fMRI), we now know that the brain is always changing in response to the environment. We can mould our brain and can even build a stronger and healthier one. We can do this throughout life by staying healthy and active both physically and mentally. In sum, our brain is "plastic".[16]

* * *

HOW ARE PHOBIAS CLASSIFIED?

Phobias have long been a topic of psychology and psychiatry. Our understanding and classification of them are a work in progress.

In 1940, a list of fears appeared in the first edition of the *Psychiatric Dictionary*.[17] This dictionary is now in its ninth edition.[18] With each subsequent edition, the list of phobias has expanded. For example, Bathmophobia (fear of thresholds) was added. At the same time, a few phobias were dropped from the list, but only a few. For example, Homilophobia (fear of sermons) was deleted. The development of this list

7

over the last 70 years indicates something about the changing nature of extreme, excessive and unreasonable fears in society.

Phobias achieved "official" diagnostic status recognition in the *Diagnostic and Statistical Manual of Mental Disorders* (DSM), published by the American Psychiatric Association, in 1952.[19] This is the guide that the mental health and legal communities use throughout the English-speaking world and beyond to define what is and what is not a mental disease or condition. The DSM is now in its fourth-edition text revision (DSM-IV-TR) and the DSM-V is scheduled to be published in 2013.[20]

In 1959, a review published by the World Health Organization (WHO) showed that phobias were recognised as having diagnostic status in the mental health community in only three of nine "official, semi-official or national classifications" of mental diseases and conditions.[21]

According to Professor Isaac Marks of the University of London, in his pioneering and remarkable book, *Fears and Phobias* (1969), "I have presented one way of classifying phobic states but there are other ways in which the clinical material could have been subdivided".[22] Marks classified all phobias into one of three large categories: 1) Social phobias (those that involve people), 2) Agoraphobia (those that involve space) and 3) Simple phobias (those that involve everything else). This classification was integrated into the DSM, where only five or six pages are routinely devoted to phobias, beginning in 1987.[23] Departing from Marks's phobia classification categories, phobias can be divided into six categories:

1) *Animal phobias* (AP) involve animals, insects and living creatures besides humans.
2) *Body phobias* (BP) involve bodily conditions, body parts, diseases, illnesses, medical procedures and treatments, and non-social behaviours.
3) *Cultural phobias* (CP) involve ideas and places. Often these have great historical, ideological, religious or social significance.

4) *Natural Phenomena phobias* (NP) involve material things and occurrences of nature.

5) *Social phobias* (SP) involve people and social behaviours.

6) *Technological phobias* (TP) involve material things invented and produced by humans.

The reader can judge whether the classification categories of this book are an improvement over Marks's.

WHAT ARE THE MOST COMMON PHOBIAS?

Early studies indicated that phobias roughly described as Agoraphobic were involved in about 50 per cent of clinical cases. Illness phobia was involved in about 15 per cent of clinical cases. Injury phobia was involved in about 10 per cent of clinical cases. Death phobia was involved in about 10 per cent of clinical cases and social phobia was involved in roughly eight per cent of clinical cases.[24]

The list of the most common phobias in order of prominence is difficult to determine, particularly as they differ somewhat in childhood compared with adulthood (see Chapter 22). Based upon years of reports, the 50 most common phobias in adulthood look something like this (in alphabetical order):

1) Aging (Aetatemophobia)
2) Alone (Being Alone) (Eremophobia)
3) Bad People (Scelerophobia)
4) Bats (Vespertiliophobia)
5) Blood (Haematophobia)
6) Bridges (Gephyrophobia)
7) Cancer (Carcinomatophobia)
8) Cats (Felinophobia)
9) Choking (Being Choked) (Pnigophobia)

10) Corpses (Necrophobia)

11) Crowds (Ochlophobia)

12) Darkness (Achluophobia)

13) Death (Thanatophobia)

14) Deformity (Dysmorphophobia)

15) Dentists (Dentophobia)

16) Disease (Nosophobia)

17) Doctors (Iatrophobia)

18) Dogs (Caninophobia)

19) Drowning (Aquaphobia)

20) Embarrassment (Sociophobia)

21) Enclosed Spaces (Claustrophobia)

22) Failure (Atychiphobia)

23) Fire (Pyrophobia)

24) Firearms (Hoplophobia)

25) Flying (Flying in an Aircraft) (Aviophobia)

26) Frogs (Ranidaphobia)

27) Germs (Spermophobia)

28) High Places (Acrophobia)

29) Injections (Trypanophobia)

30) Insects (Entomophobia)

31) Lightning (Keraunophobia)

32) Mirrors (Eisoptrophobia)

33) Monitored (Being Monitored) (Monitorphobia)

34) Pain (One's Own) (Algophobia)

35) Pointed Objects (Aichmophobia)

36) Police (Policiophobia)

37) Public Places (Agoraphobia)

38) Public Speaking (Glossophobia)

39) Rats (Rodentophobia)

40) Rejection (Including by Peers) (Rejectuphobia)

41) Reptiles (Herpetophobia)

42) Ridicule (Catagelophobia)

43) Sharks (Selachophobia)

44) Snakes (Ophidiophobia)

45) Social Situations (Sociophobia)

46) Spiders (Arachnophobia)

47) Terrorism (Terror-phobia)

48) Thunder (Brontophobia)

49) Uncleanliness (Rhypophobia)

50) Vomiting (Emetophobia)

WHAT ARE THE STRANGEST PHOBIAS?

A rule among humans is that what is familiar behaviour to someone is strange behaviour to someone else. "Strange" is used here in the sense of what is uncommon. A morbid fear of high places (Acrophobia) is certainly more commonly found among humans than a morbid fear of teddy bears (Archtophobia). It is a matter of statistics and not one of moral judgement. Nevertheless, if someone is fearful of teddy bears and not of high places, they suffer in the same way as someone who fears high places and not teddy bears. Having a strange phobia can no doubt make you feel lonely. Saying someone has a strange phobia in no way denigrates the person for having this phobia nor does it detract from the impact the strange phobia has upon a person's life. What is a strange phobia is pretty much in the eye of the beholder. A long list of phobias is included in this book. Undoubtedly some of these phobias will be regarded by many, if not most, readers as strange. The reader may make this judgement, hopefully with a sense of understanding and compassion.

HOW ARE PHOBIAS TREATED?

Chapter 21 covers the treatment of phobias. Treatment is not a focus of this book. It is not within the competence of the author, as an anthropologist, to diagnose and treat; treatment should be performed by a licensed mental health professional and clinician. Nevertheless, it can be reported that mental health professionals say that a phobia is the easiest and quickest mental condition to treat. Phobia and anxiety clinics exist in major cities and elsewhere for this purpose. Most therapies rely upon cognitive behavioural therapy (CBT) or variations of CBT. In addition, eye-movement therapy, hypnotherapy and antidepressant medications can be utilised.

WHERE IN THE BRAIN ARE PHOBIAS STORED?

Central physiological mechanisms underlying phobias and fears are largely situated in deep brain structures, such as the hypothalamus, amygdala and other parts of the limbic system. However, different aspects of fearful behaviour depend upon separate but interlinked central mechanisms. The amygdala is an area of the brain located behind the pituitary gland. The amygdala may trigger the secretion of hormones that affect fear and aggression. When the fear or aggression response is initiated, the amygdala may also trigger the release of hormones to help put the body into an "alert" state, the so-called "fight-or-flight".[25]

WHAT HAPPENS TO THE BODY WHEN EXPERIENCING A PHOBIA?

When you experience a phobia, an intense fear sets your body in motion so it's ready to deal with any threat. This is what happens in the body and sometimes the consequences can be long-term:

- *Eyes:* Fight-or-flight hormones, like norepinephrine, dilate pupils to improve vision.
- *Heart:* The heart pumps faster, increasing blood pressure to accelerate the delivery of oxygen. Prolonged high blood pressure increases risk of heart attack or stroke.

- *Lungs:* Breathing rate increases as lungs take in more oxygen. Long-term stress responses exacerbate conditions such as asthma and hyperventilation that can trigger a panic attack.
- *Skin:* Sweat glands start working to cool the body down. But long-term stress can suppress wound healing, making the body prone to infection.
- *Hormones:* The adrenal glands secrete cortisol, a stress hormone. Too much cortisol corrodes bones and muscles, can weaken the immune system, and thus diminishes at least some immune response.
- *Stomach:* The stomach stops digesting so the body can divert energy elsewhere in the body. Slow digestion may result in an increase in stomach acid and cause nausea or inflame a stomach ulcer.
- *Intestines:* During a stress response, blood is shunted away from the intestines, suppressing digestion. Continually suppressed digestion can trigger irritable bowel syndrome.[26]

* * *

PHOBIAS LINKED TO PHYSICAL CONDITIONS

Phobias, as well as anxiety disorders, generally appear to be independently associated with several physical conditions, including thyroid disease, respiratory disease, arthritis and migraine headaches. This is according to a study of 4,181 adults by a team of Canadian researchers led by Dr Jitender Sareen. The researchers argue that this co-occurrence of disorders may significantly increase the risk of disability and negatively affect quality of life. Although depression has long been linked to physical illness, evidence supporting an association between phobias, anxiety disorders generally and physical health problems is more recent. The researchers point out that "studies have found that those with phobic (fearful) anxiety may be more likely to experience sudden cardiac death, and rates of anxiety disorders are higher than expected in patients with thyroid disease, cancer, hypertension and several other conditions".[27]

* * *

IS THERE A SINGLE THEORY FOR PHOBIAS AND FEARS?

No single theory accounts for all the ways in which phobias and fears are learned. Phobias and fears can be learned easily as a response to previously neutral stimuli. Fears have a foundation in biology and are useful in survival. Fear is a drive that motivates the learning and performance of new responses in the same way as hunger, thirst and other drives. Experimental paradigms of fear include classical conditioning situations, avoidance and escape conditioning, temporal pacing and punishment training.

ARE THERE SEX DIFFERENCES IN PHOBIAS?

Before puberty, both sexes seem equally susceptible to most fears. After puberty, women seem to be more susceptible to most phobias. There are hardly any phobias that men consistently experience more often than women, apart from those phobias that can only be experienced by men.

WHAT PERCENTAGE OF THE POPULATION SUFFERS FROM A PHOBIA?

It may be impossible to determine for sure the percentage of phobics in the population. One early US study estimated that 7.7 per cent of the general population suffered from a phobia, while severely disabling phobias characterised only 0.22 per cent. It was also found that less than 0.1 per cent was receiving psychiatric treatment for a phobia but that 0.9 per cent had treatment at some time for a phobia.

DOES AGE MATTER IN PHOBIA STIMULI?

Certain classes of stimuli are more likely to trigger phobias at particular ages, regardless of the frequency of exposure to such stimuli. Sudden loud noises or movements trigger fear easily in very young infants. Fear of strangers is the rule in older infants. Fear of animals usually begins in preschool-aged children. Fear of open spaces and social situations starts later and is rare in childhood.[28]

DO WE INHERIT THE PHOBIAS OF OUR PARENTS?

It has been known since the 1930s that a high correlation exists between phobias reported by the mother and those reported by the child. This figure may be as high as 67 per cent. The father does not seem to be as important in this "carrier" role.[29]

DOES A PHOBIA LAST FOR A LIFETIME?

A little less than 13 per cent of phobias remains with the sufferer their entire life. At least this was the case for 2,064 young German women involved in the Dresden Mental Health Study. A team of seven doctors led by Dr Eni S. Becker of the Behavioural Science Institute of Radboud University in Nijmegen, the Netherlands, writes that "the lifetime prevalence of any specific phobia was 12.8 per cent, with subtypes ranging in prevalence between 0.2 per cent (vomiting, infections) and five per cent (animals)". The researchers add that "specific phobias are common among young women", but that they differ in prevalence, depending upon the age at which they begin and if another condition occurs with it (co-morbidity).[30]

WHAT IS A PANIC ATTACK?

Phobias and fears can show themselves in the form of "panic attacks". About six per cent of people suffer from panic attacks. The condition is more properly called panic disorder. The major symptom of a panic attack is a sudden wave of terror that can strike anytime, anywhere, and for no apparent reason. During an attack, a person may experience heart palpitations, chest pains, shortness of breath, gasping for air, smothering sensations, feelings of being choked, faintness, sweating, shaking, nausea, cramping, dizziness, tingling or numbing sensations in the hands, chills, hot flushes, horrible foreboding, even out-of-body sensations. Sufferers may think they are dying or going mad. Yet the level of fear is totally out of proportion to the actual situation. A few things that we know about panic disorder include:

- An attack passes in a few minutes. The body's "panic" response cannot hold up for much longer than that.
- Although some people have just one attack and never experience another, other people suffer attacks daily, and still others have up to 10 per day.
- Those leading anxiety-filled lives are the most at risk.
- Attacks generally strike during periods of high stress.
- Some of the most common triggers of an attack are the death of someone very close, the loss of a significant relationship, the birth of a child, hospitalisation, moving home and job-related stress.
- Most panic disorder sufferers share the characteristic of worrying a great deal about everyday matters. They often are overly concerned about what others think of them, bottle up their feelings, never feel competent, see everything in terms of "black" and "white", are perfectionists, highly emotional, very conscientious and tend to take on the problems of others.
- The worst sufferers of panic disorder have as much as a 20 times greater chance of attempting suicide.
- Panic disorder tends to run in families. This suggests a genetic component involved in its cause.
- If one identical twin has panic disorder, there is a 30 per cent chance that the other twin will have it too.
- Medications control symptoms in about 90 per cent of patients.

Chapter 2
Phobias Starting with A

"To suffering there is a limit; to fearing, none."
Sir Francis Bacon (1561–1626), *Essays*, "Of Seditions and Troubles"

If something exists, there is someone, somewhere, who is deathly afraid of it. That is the reality of phobias.

Our journey through this fascinating world of our deepest fears logically enough starts with those abnormal, morbid, persistent and unreasonable fears beginning with the letter "A" and continues through to those beginning with the letter "Z". For each, the phobic stimulus is listed alphabetically, followed by the phobia name and then the classification of the phobia into one of six categories: 1) Animal phobias (AP), 2) Body phobias (BP), 3) Cultural phobias (CP), 4) Natural Phenomena phobias (NP), 5) Social phobias (SP) or 6) Technological phobias (TP). The phobia name is based upon the etymology of the, usually Greek or Latin, root. When a "less preferred" term is listed, it is less preferred for this particular phobia but may be the preferred term for a different phobia. It may also be listed as "less preferred" due to variation in spelling from the preferred term. Other aspects of the phobia are mentioned, including anecdotes about it, the famous who may suffer from it and the odd summary of a research study pertaining to that phobia. Please note that internet sources have been utilised for celebrities in particular. The author takes some of these sources with a grain of salt — as should the reader.

ABANDONMENT

Abannumaphobia (SP) — From Latin *bannum* meaning "to give up absolutely (as in control)". This includes fear of left behind (being left behind). Abandonment and falling are the two basic fears of infants, especially abandonment. Fear of falling seems to decline after age one or so. Not so abandonment. Fear of abandonment occurs before the fear of death — before even the concept of death. It is the most powerful reason for infant crying, and something from which many of us never recover.

Case: A 63-year-old woman has been afraid of being abandoned her entire life. "I have suffered great loss throughout my life. Many people close to me have died. I know that one day I will be alone. I think about this always. I was afraid of being abandoned when I was a little girl. It is never far from my thoughts."[1]

ABORTION

Abortivuphobia (BP) — From Latin *abortivus* meaning "causing abortion". This includes fear of miscarriage.

ABUSE

Agraphobia (SP) — From Greek *agra* meaning "seizing or catching".

ACCIDENTS

Dystychiphobia (NP) — From Greek *dys* meaning "bad or harsh" and *tyche* meaning "luck". This includes fear of bad luck.

ACCOUNTABILITY

See Responsibility — Hypengyophobia.

ACCULTURATION

Acculturaphobia (CP) — From Latin *cultura* meaning "tend, guard, cultivate or till". This includes fear of assimilation.

ACID DEW

See Acid Rain — Acidusrigarephobia.

ACID RAIN

Acidusrigarephobia (NP) — From Latin *acidus* meaning "sour" and *rigare* meaning "to wet". This includes fear of acid dew.

ACTING

See Stage (The Stage) — Topophobia.

ACTION

See Work — Ergasiophobia.

ACUPUNCTURE

Acusapungerephobia (BP) — From Latin *acus* meaning "needle" and *pungere* meaning "to prick or pierce".

ADDICTION

Addicerophobia (BP) — From Latin *addicere* meaning "to deliver, yield or devote".

Case: "I stay away from things that are bad for me because I really fear addiction. I have an addictive personality. Once I start, I can't stop."

ADDRESSES

See Sermons — Homilophobia.

ADOLESCENT FEMALES

Nymphophobia (SP) — From Greek *nymphe* meaning "adolescent female". The opposite of this phobia is Nymphophilia, the sexual attraction to female adolescents.

ADOLESCENT MALES

Ephebophobia (SP) — From Latin *ephebos* meaning "adolescent boy". A less preferred term is Ephebiophobia. The opposite of this phobia is Ephebophilia, the sexual attraction to male adolescents.

AEROPLANES

See Flying (Flying in an Aircraft) — Aviophobia.

AFRAID (BEING AFRAID)

See Fears — Phobophobia.

AFRICA (THINGS AFRICAN)

Afrophobia (CP) — From Latin *Africa* meaning "the land of Africa".

AGE DIFFERENCES

See Time — Chronophobia.

AGING

Aetatemophobia (BP) — From Greek *aetatem* meaning "period of life". Less preferred terms are Gerascophobia and Gerontophobia. If you are an Aetatemophobe, you share this with US model and actress Jessica Biel. Biel "admits that she is terrified of aging and wrinkles" and has obsessive thoughts about it. There are, no doubt, many who work before the camera who also experience this dread of aging. But as the old saying goes, "Aging is the one thing of which no one wants to be cured".

Case: A 79-year-old woman says, "I was always afraid of getting old. I still am. Now that I really am old, I have to live with the fear of getting older. The fear of the loss of memory from old age is the worst and being a burden to other people too. Getting old is the toughest thing I've ever done."[2]

AIDS

AIDS-phobia (BP) — From modern terms, "AIDS" is an acronym for the medical condition of acquired immune deficiency syndrome. This includes fear of HIV.

Case: "I'm so afraid of catching AIDS that I never have sex — protected or not."

AIR

Aerophobia (NP) — From Greek *aer* meaning "air". This includes fear of air swallowing. A less preferred term is Anemophobia.

* * *

AEROPHOBIA AND RABIES
In 2004 in Mexico, a male patient died of rabies after being bitten by a sick bat. The patient experienced the usual intense fear of water (rabies in humans is called hydrophobia to indicate the major symptom). The patient also experienced an intense fear of air. The doctor reporting on this patient claimed that less well-known, even among the medical profession, is the fact that such patients also fear air.[3]

* * *

AIR DRAUGHTS
See Wind — Anemophobia.

AIR POLLUTION
Aeropolluerephobia (NP) — From Greek *aer* meaning "air" and *polluere* meaning "to soil, defile or contaminate". This includes fear of airborne noxious substances.

AIR SICKNESS
Aeronausiphobia (BP) — From Greek *aer* meaning "air" and *naus* meaning "ship". This includes fear of vomiting due to air sickness.

AIR SWALLOWING
See Air — Aerophobia.

AIRBORNE NOXIOUS SUBSTANCES
See Air Pollution — Aeropolluerephobia.

AIRCRAFT
See Flying (Flying in an Aircraft) — Aviophobia.

ALCOHOL
Methylphobia (NP) — From Greek *methyl* meaning "alcohol". This includes fear of alcoholic (being or becoming an alcoholic),

drunkenness and intoxication. Less preferred terms are Dipsophobia and Potophobia. Famed US pioneer physician and "father of American psychiatry" Dr Benjamin Rush (1745–1813) wrote of five cases of what he referred to as "rum phobia". But what Rush seems to have been describing is an allergy to rum.[4]

ALCOHOLIC (BEING OR BECOMING AN ALCOHOLIC)

See Alcohol — Methylphobia.

ALL THINGS

Panphobia (NP) — From Greek *pan* meaning "all". This includes fear of anything. Less preferred terms are Pamphobia, Panophobia and Pantophobia. Pan, the Greek god of flocks, pastures and wood, was believed by the ancient Greeks to be the source of all fears.

ALLIGATORS

See Reptiles — Herpetophobia.

ALONE (BEING ALONE)

Eremophobia (SP) — From Greek *eremos* meaning "a desert". This includes fear of desolate places, deserted places, isolation, loneliness, lost (being lost), oneself (being by oneself), solitude and stillness. Less preferred terms are Agoraphobia, Autophobia, Eremiophobia, Eremiphobia, Ermitophobia, Insulaphobia, Isolophobia, Monophobia and Phobophobia. If you are an Eremophobe, you share this with the great German poet, novelist and playwright Johann Wolfgang von Goethe. Goethe was terrified of being alone and always sought people to be around him. Dr Benjamin Rush called this phobia "solo phobia" and was contemptuous of it. He wrote: "This distemper is peculiar to persons of vacant minds and guilty consciences. Such people cannot bear to be alone, especially if the horror of sickness is added to the pain of attempting to think, or to the terror of thinking." When Rush wrote this, he was obviously not thinking of Goethe.

The mind of the creator of *Faust* was anything but vacant. French actress Brigitte Bardot said of herself: "Solitude scares me. It makes me think about love, death and war. I need distraction from anxious, black thoughts."

Case: "I don't know why, but as far back as I can remember I have been terrified of being alone. The idea of dying alone is my greatest fear of all."[5]

AMERICA (THINGS AMERICAN)

Ameriphobia (CP) — From Latin *Americanus* meaning "the land of America". Less preferred terms are Amerophobia and Columbophobia.

AMNESIA

Amnesiophobia (BP) — From Greek *amnesia* meaning "oblivion". This includes fear of forgetfulness and memory loss. A less preferred term is Amnesiphobia.

AMPHIBIANS (ANYTHING AMPHIBIOUS)

Batrachophobia (AP) — From Greek *batrachos* meaning "amphibians". Less preferred terms are Bufonophobia, Pleurodeliphobia, Ranidaphobia and Urodelaphobia.

AMPUTATIONS

Apotemnophobia (BP) — From Greek *apo* meaning "away from" and *temnein* meaning "to cut". This includes fear of losing a body part. The opposite of this phobia is Apotemnophilia, the sexual attraction to losing a limb or being an amputee.

AMPUTEES

Acrotomophobia (SP) — From Greek *acron* meaning "extremity" and *temnein* meaning "to cut". The opposite of this phobia is Acrotomophilia, the sexual attraction to amputees.

Case: "People with missing parts. That's what I'm afraid of."

ANALGESICS (PAINKILLERS)

See Medicines — Pharmacophobia.

ANGELS

See Spectres — Spectrophobia.

ANGER

Angrophobia (SP) — From Latin *angere* meaning "to throttle or torment". A less preferred term is Cholerophobia.

ANGER (ANOTHER'S)

Cholerophobia (SP) — From Latin *chole* meaning "bile" (as in filled with a toxic substance). This includes fear of angry people.

ANGINA

See Heart Disease — Cardiopathophobia.

ANGRY PEOPLE

See Anger (Another's) — Cholerophobia.

ANIMAL SKINS AND FUR

Doraphobia (AP) — From Greek *dora* meaning "skin or hide". This includes fear of fur and leather. The opposite of this phobia is Doraphilia, the sexual attraction to animal skins and fur, including leather, or sexual activity involving animal skins and fur, including leather products.

ANIMALS (DOMESTIC)

Zoophobia (AP) — From Greek *zoion* meaning "animal". A less preferred term is Agrizoophobia. The opposite of this phobia is Zoophilia, the sexual attraction to animals. Odder still, the sexual attraction to animals trained for sex is Androgynozoophilia. Zoophobia is fear of animals in general. Fear of a particular species of animal is the phobia for that animal. Among the most common animal phobias are bees, birds, cats, dogs, fish, frogs, horses, insects, mice, rabbits, rats, sharks, snakes and spiders. A real or imagined frightening experience with the animal is the source of the zoophobia. Often a phobia of one animal is generalised to a similar animal or even to all animals. Although most zoophobias develop between the ages of four and eight, if an individual experiences a traumatic event involving an animal (for instance, being bitten by a dog), the phobia can develop in late childhood, in adolescence or in adulthood. Sigmund Freud theorised that an animal phobia is the displacement of the child's fear from a person important in their emotional life onto some animal selected by the child according to their childhood experiences. This could be a wolf, a lion, a snake and so on. The animal becomes the substitute for the feared person. The advantage to the person is that they can avoid their anxiety by avoiding the animal. Unlike the Freudians, behaviourists tend to emphasise the learned nature of animal fears either from direct traumatic exposure (classical conditioning) or from vicarious observation (for instance, seeing someone attacked by the animal, watching the films *Jaws* and *Arachnophobia*, etc.). It is interesting to note that 95 per cent of those with zoophobia are female.[6]

ANIMALS (WILD)

Agrizoophobia (AP) — From Latin *agri* meaning "field" and Greek *zoion* meaning "animal". This includes fear of wild animals. A less preferred term is Zoophobia.

ANIMATED CHARACTERS

Animatuphobia (TP) — From Latin *animatus* meaning "give breath to". This includes fear of cartoons. If you are an Animatuphobe, you share this with US–Israeli actress Natalie Portman. Portman is allegedly afraid of the Smurfs cartoon characters. According to one report, "The little blue things really creep her out".[7]

ANIMATRONIC CREATURES

Automatonophobia (AP) — From Greek *automato* meaning "driven from inside oneself". The first animatronic creature to feature in a movie was the giant squid in Walt Disney's *20,000 Leagues Under The Sea* in 1954. Disney introduced animatronic creations of various sorts in his Disneyland theme park, which opened about the same time (18 July 1955). Although by the end of 2009 some 600 million people had visited Disneyland to have fun, for an Automatonophobe Disneyland would be a chamber of horrors.

ANTELOPE

See Deer — Alkephobia.

ANTIDEPRESSANTS

See Medicines — Pharmacophobia.

ANTIQUES

Antiquphobia (TP) — From Latin *antiquus* meaning "old, ancient or former". US actor, director and writer Billy Bob Thornton supposedly suffers from this phobia. According to one report, Thornton refuses to stay in a room with furniture built before 1950, saying, "I get creeped out and can't breathe and I can't eat around it". According to another report, he says, "I just don't like old stuff. I'm creeped out by it, and I have no explanation why ... I don't have a phobia about American antiques, it's mostly French — you know, like the big, old, gold-carved chairs with the velvet cushions. The Louis XIV type. That's what creeps me out. I can spot the imitation antiques a mile off. They have a different vibe. Not as much dust. I won't use real silver. You know, like the big, old, heavy-ass forks and knives, I can't do that. Pieces from 1700 and 1800 France and England really freak me out, especially harpsichords."[8]

ANTS

Formicaphobia (AP) — From Latin *formica* meaning "ant". A less preferred term is Myrmecophobia. The opposite of this phobia is Formicophilia, the sexual attraction to ants.

Case: An 89-year-old woman says, "A long time ago when I was just a girl, I placed a cake I had made on a blanket at a picnic. In what seemed only a few minutes, ants were all over it. I was horrified. I cried. I still cringe at the memory. I have been afraid of ants ever since. I'm afraid that ants will be in my mouth and stomach. Somehow they will get to my food after I've eaten it just as they got to my cake."

ANUS (THE ANUS)

See Rectum — Proctophobia.

ANYTHING

See All Things — Panphobia.

APES

Primatephobia (AP) — From Latin *primas* meaning "of the first rank, chief or principal". This includes fear of monkeys and non-human primates. Less preferred terms are Maimouphobia and Pithikosophobia.

APOCALYPSE (THE APOCALYPSE)

Apocalypsiphobia (CP) — From Greek *apokayptein* meaning "uncovering or revelation". This includes fear of the end of the world. A less preferred term is Cosmophobia.

APPLAUSE

See Approval — Approbarephobia.

APPROVAL

Approbarephobia (SP) — From Latin *approbare* meaning "to assent to as good, regard as good". This includes fear of applause

and praise. Less preferred terms are Alloxodoxaphobia and
Doxophobia.

ARCHES

Arcusaphobia (TP) — From Latin *arcus* meaning "arc, arch or
bow".

ARRHYTHMIA

See Heart Disease — Cardiopathophobia.

ARSON

Arsonphobia (SP) — From Latin *arsionem* meaning "a burning".

ASIA (THINGS ASIAN)

Asiaphobia (CP) — From Greek *Asia* meaning "the land from
which the sun rises".

ASPERGER'S SYNDROME

See Autism — Autism-phobia.

ASSIMILATION

See Acculturation — Acculturaphobia.

ASTHMA

See Chronic Obstructive Pulmonary Disease — COPD-phobia.

ASTROLOGERS

See Astrology — Astrologiaphobia.

ASTROLOGY

Astrologiaphobia (CP) — From Greek *astrologia* meaning "telling
of the stars". This includes fear of astrologers.

ASYMMETRY

Asymmetriphobia (NP) — From Greek *symmetros* meaning
"symmetry, evenness or proportionality".

ATAXIA

Ataxiaphobia (BP) — From Greek *a* meaning "not" and *taxis* meaning "order". This includes fear of muscular uncoordination. Less preferred terms are Ataxiophobia and Ataxophobia. Ataxia is a medical condition characterised by a debilitating lack of coordination of muscle movements.

ATHLETIC CONTESTS

See Sports — Sports-phobia.

ATOMIC DISASTERS

See Atomic Energy and Science — Atomosophobia.

ATOMIC ENERGY AND SCIENCE

Atomosophobia (TP) — From Greek *atomos* meaning "uncut and indivisible". This includes fear of atomic disasters, atomic explosions, atomic power plants, atomic wars, atomic weapons, nuclear disasters, nuclear energy and science, nuclear explosions, nuclear power plants, nuclear wars and nuclear weapons. A less preferred term is Nucleomituphobia.

ATOMIC EXPLOSIONS

See Atomic Energy and Science — Atomosophobia.

ATOMIC POWER PLANTS

See Atomic Energy and Science — Atomosophobia.

ATOMIC WARS

See Atomic Energy and Science — Atomosophobia.

ATOMIC WEAPONS

See Atomic Energy and Science — Atomosophobia.

ATTENTION

See Social Situations — Sociophobia.

AUDITORIUMS

See Theatres — Theatrophobia.

AURORA AUSTRALIS

See Auroras — Auroraphobia.

AURORA BOREALIS

See Auroras — Auroraphobia.

AURORAS

Auroraphobia (NP) — From Latin *aurora* meaning "dawn". This includes fear of aurora australis, aurora borealis, northern lights and southern lights. Aurora was the Roman goddess of the dawn. In the southern latitudes, the polar light is the aurora australis (from Latin *Australis* meaning "southern land"). While in the northern latitudes, the polar light is the aurora borealis (from Greek *boreas* meaning "north wind").

AUSTRALIA (THINGS AUSTRALIAN)

Australophobia (CP) — From Latin *Australis* meaning "southern land". A less preferred term is Novahollandiaphobia.

AUTHORITY

Auctoritaphobia (SP) — From Latin *auctoritas* meaning "command and influence".

AUTISM

Autism-phobia (BP) — From Greek *autos* meaning "self" and *ismos* meaning "action or state". This includes fear of Asperger's syndrome and Tourette's syndrome. Autism is a medical condition characterised by impaired social communication and interaction often with repetitive behaviours. Along with autism itself, Asperger's syndrome and Tourette's syndrome are known together as autism spectrum disorder.

AUTISM SPECTRUM DISORDER

See Autism — Autism-phobia.

AUTOMOBILES

See Cars — Autokinetophobia.

AUTOMOBILES (BEING A PASSENGER IN AN AUTOMOBILE)

See Cars (Being a Passenger in a Car) — Motorphobia.

AUTOMOBILES (DRIVING AN AUTOMOBILE)

See Cars (Driving a Car) — Mobilophobia.

AWARD CEREMONIES

See Ceremonies — Teleophobia.

Chapter 3
Phobias Starting with B

"The oldest and strongest emotion of mankind is fear."

H.P. Lovecraft (1890–1937), *Supernatural Horror in Literature*

BABIES

See **Infants** — Infantiphobia.

BACILLI

Bacillophobia (AP) — From Latin *bacillus* meaning "a little rod or stick". This includes fear of microbes and microorganisms. A less preferred term is Microbiophobia. Bacilli are a class of rod-shaped microorganisms. People often fear bacilli because some cause infections and can be seen only under a microscope or magnifying glass, so take on a mysterious quality. Only a few bacilli are actually dangerous. These are pathogens. But this does not stop a bacillophobe from being terrified of all bacilli. Many such phobics have compulsions about hand-washing and cleanliness. Others are obsessively concerned about or fearful of germs (Spermophobia).

BACTERIA

Bacteriophobia (AP) — From Greek *bakterion* meaning "a little stick".

BAD BREATH

Halitophobia (BP) — From Latin *halitus* meaning "breath".

Case: "Bad breath is my greatest fear. I hate it. I'm always checking my breath. I do this at least 100 times per day. I don't eat a lot of things that give you bad breath. I hate it on others too. It's disgusting. I have nightmares of a disgusting old man breathing on me with really bad breath."

BAD DREAMS

See Dreams — Oneirophobia.

BAD LUCK

See Accidents — Dystychiphobia.

BAD NEWS

Dysphophobia (CP) — From Greek *dysphoria* meaning "depression". This includes fear of hearing bad news.

BAD PEOPLE

Scelerophobia (SP) — From Latin *sceleris* meaning "a crime, wickedness or evil deed". This includes fear of burglars, harm (being harmed by bad people), kidnappers, muggers, murderers, robbers, thieves and wicked people. An older and quaint Latin expression for this phobia is *pavor sceleris* meaning "quaking in the presence of evil". *Pavor* in Latin roughly translates to "afraid, terrified or repulsed". In war zones, high civil unrest regions or high crime areas, such fears are reasonable and individuals may take legitimate precautions. However, when these fears are out of balance with the degree of danger and when unreasonable precautions restrict the normal activities of a person, then the fear crosses the line and becomes a phobia. In children, *pavor diurnus* is the angst experienced right after the afternoon nap (*diurnus* means "daytime") and *pavor nocturnus* is the angst experienced during the night (*nocturnus* means "night-time"). Sometimes the latter is called night terrors, sleep terrors or sleep terror disorder. US actor, director, writer and comedian Woody Allen is a Scelerophobe, according to English psychologist and author Dr Oliver James. Allen is supposedly terrified of bad people and especially of being kidnapped by them.

Case: "Oh, and [serial killer] Richard Speck. I don't know if you know who he is, but he is a mass murderer from the 1970s that killed a group of nurses. He makes me sick to my stomach and I have a fear of seeing his image. He makes me want to vomit."[1]

BADGERS

See Weasels — Galeophobia.

BALANCE (BEING BALANCED)

Librophobia (BP) — From Latin *libra* meaning "balance, scale or unit of weight".

BALD (BEING OR BECOMING BALD)

Phalacrophobia (BP) — From Greek *phalakros* meaning "bald-headed". This includes fear of going bald. A less preferred term is Peladophobia. US actor Tom Cruise may be a Phalacrophobe. According to one report, Cruise is supposedly so afraid of going bald that "the actor counts every hair that comes out". But perhaps he gives them away as souvenirs to his adoring fans.[2]

BALD PEOPLE

Peladophobia (SP) — From Greek *pella* meaning "stone" and implying smoothness. A less preferred term is Phalacrophobia.

BALLOONS

Pallonophobia (TP) — From Latin *pallone* meaning "large ball". A less preferred term is Globaphobia. If you are a Pallonophobe, you share this with famed English film director Alfred Hitchcock and English model and TV personality Charlotte Mears. Mears says that she cannot stand balloons: "I've been scared of balloons for as long as I can possibly remember. I've always hated going to parties because of the sight of other people holding balloons and the anticipation of them popping."

Case: "I'm terrified of balloons. I will scream and go into shock if confronted by a balloon, particularly in the hands of children. All my life I have been tormented by and because of balloons."[3]

BANANAS

Bananaphobia (NP) — From Wolof (West Africa) *banana* meaning "banana". The ancient Greeks and Romans did not eat bananas so did not have a word for it.

BANK PASSWORDS

See Passwords — Friend-or-phobia.

BANKS

See Money — Chrematophobia.

BARBED WIRE

See Fences — Clauderephobia.

BARBER SHOPS

See Barbers — Barbaphobia.

BARBER'S POLES

See Barbers — Barbaphobia.

BARBERS

Barbaphobia (SP) — From Latin *barba* meaning "beard". This includes fear of barber shops, barber's poles and haircuts. A less preferred term is Tonsurephobia. German philosopher Arthur Schopenhauer was a Barbaphobe, according to two psychologists. Schopenhauer, the champion of "blind will" as a personal ideal that empowered the individual to overcome all obstacles and fears, was evidently terrified of his own barber.[4]

BARLEY

Barleyphobia (NP) — From Latin *bar* meaning "coarse, grain meal".

BARREN SPACES

Kenophobia (NP) — From Latin *kenos* meaning "empty".
This includes fear of emptiness, empty rooms, empty spaces,
vacuums and voids. Less preferred terms are Cenophobia and
Centophobia.

BATHING (DROWNING)

See Drowning — Aquaphobia.

BATHING (WASHING)

See Washing — Ablutophobia.

BATHROOMS (PRIVATE)

See Washing — Ablutophobia.

BATHROOMS (PUBLIC)

See Lavatories — Lavatoriphobia.

BATS

Vespertiliophobia (AP) — From Latin *vespertillio* meaning
"bat" and implying "of the evening or night". If you are a
Vespertiliophobe, you share this with famed English writer Charles
Dickens and English singer Gareth Gates.

Case: A 48-year-old woman says, "I hate fruit bats. I won't
go out at night unless I can stay in a car. I hear them in the trees
and flying around and am sure they're going to swoop on me. I
don't like magpies for the same reason but at least I can see them.
Magpies in the day, fruit bats at night."[5]

BEARDS

Pogonophobia (SP) — From Greek *pogon* meaning "a beard".
A less preferred term is Pognophobia. In one of his classic
experiments in stimulus-response conditioning, John Watson, the
famous US psychologist and "father of behaviourism", was able to
induce Pogonophobia by conditioning a young boy to be afraid of

beards. Whenever the boy saw a beard, Watson rang a deafeningly loud bell. The boy became traumatised. This would be regarded as a highly unethical experiment today.

BEARING A DEFORMED CHILD
See Deformed Children — Teratophobia.

BEARING A MONSTER
See Deformed Children — Teratophobia.

BEARS
Ursuphobia (AP) — From Latin *ursus* meaning "bear".

BEATEN IN PRIVATE (BEING BEATEN IN PRIVATE)
Rhabdophobia (SP) — From Greek *rhabdos* meaning "a rod". This includes fear of caned (being caned in private), flogged (being flogged in private), magic wands, punished (being punished in private), rods, scourged (being scourged in private), spanked (being spanked in private), sticks and whipped (being whipped in private). Less preferred terms are Mastigophobia and Poinephobia. The opposite of this phobia is Rhabdophilia, the sexual attraction to being beaten, caned, flogged, scourged, spanked or whipped in private.

BEATEN IN PUBLIC (BEING BEATEN IN PUBLIC)
Mastigophobia (SP) — From Greek *mastix* meaning "whipped". This includes fear of caned (being caned in public), flogged (being flogged in public), punished (being punished in public), scourged (being scourged in public), spanked (being spanked in public) and whipped (being whipped in public). Less preferred terms are Poinephobia and Rhabdophobia.[6]

BEATING ONESELF
Battuerephobia (BP) — From Latin *battuere* meaning "to beat".

BEAUTIFUL MEN (HANDSOME MEN)

Caliandrophobia (SP) — From Greek *cali* meaning "beautiful" and *andros* meaning "men".

BEAUTIFUL WOMEN (HANDSOME WOMEN)

Caligynephobia (SP) — From Greek *cali* meaning "beautiful" and *gyne* meaning "women". Less preferred terms are Gynephobia, Gynophobia and Venustraphobia.

BEAUTY SALONS

Bellusaphobia (SP) — From Latin *bellus* meaning "beautiful or fine". It can refer to fear of judgements of others as to one's beauty, chemicals placed upon the head, confinement in the chair, temporary appearance while not at one's best, and other things associated with beauty salons.

BED-WETTING

Eneuresisophobia (BP) — From Greek *eneurein* meaning "to urinate". Eneuresis is the medical term for bed-wetting.

BEDS

Clinophobia (TP) — From Greek *klino* meaning "bed". This includes fear of bedspreads, going to bed, mattresses and pillows.

Case: A 59-year-old woman has been terrified of beds all her life. A furniture store is a nightmare for her. Going on holiday and staying in a bed in a hotel is impossible. She sleeps on a mat in her own home. After years of psychotherapy, she believes that the origin of this phobia stems from when she was a baby. She was wrapped tightly in blankets and left on top of a bed. She somehow rolled over onto her face and nearly suffocated. She says she can still see the white bedspread up close and remember how she struggled for breath.

BEDSPREADS

See Beds — Clinophobia.

BEE STINGS

See Bees — Melissaphobia.

BEES

Melissaphobia (AP) — From Greek *melissa* meaning "a bee". This includes fear of bee stings. Less preferred terms are Apiphobia and Melissophobia. The opposite of this phobia is Melissaphilia, the sexual attraction to bees or bee stings.

BEGGARS

Mendicarephobia (SP) — From Latin *mendicare* meaning "to beg". This includes fear of bums, dislocated people, dispossessed people, hobos, homeless people, itinerants, poverty (another's), tramps and vagrants. A less preferred term is Hobophobia. "Hobo" is a term from the 19th century American West, where "Ho boy" was a call to railroad workers, many of whom were itinerant.

BEHAVIOUR

See Work — Ergasiophobia.

BELCHING

Eructaphobia (BP) — From Latin *eructatio* meaning "belching".

BENDS (THE BENDS)

Aeroemphysemaphobia (BP) — From Greek *aer* meaning "air" and *emphysema* meaning "swelling". Aeroemphysema is a medical condition also known as caisson disease, decompression sickness or, more familiarly, the bends.

BEREAVEMENT

Gravarephobia (SP) — From Latin *gravare* meaning "to grieve, make heavy or be weighty (as in mourning)".

BEYOND (THE BEYOND)

Metathesiophobia (NP) — From Greek *meta* meaning "beyond" and *thesi* meaning "place".

BICYCLES

Cyclophobia (TP) — From Greek *kyklos* meaning "a wheel".

BIG OBJECTS AND THINGS

Grossusophobia (NP) — From Latin *grossus* meaning "thick or coarse". This includes fear of growing.

BIRD (BEING OR BECOMING A BIRD)

Avidsophobia (BP) — From Latin *avis* meaning "bird". The opposite of this phobia is Avidsophilia, the sexual attraction to birds.

BIRDS

Ornithophobia (AP) — From Greek *ornis* meaning "bird". If you are an Ornithophobe, you share this with English soccer star David Beckham.[7]

BIRTHDAYS

Natalisophobia (BP) — From Latin *natalia* meaning "birthday".

BITTERNESS

Amaruphobia (NP) — From Latin *amarus* meaning "bitter".

BLACK (COLOUR OR WORD)

Melanophobia (NP) — From Greek *melas* meaning "black or dark". A less preferred term is Blakphobia.

BLACK CATS

Negrofelinophobia (AP) — From Latin *nigrum* meaning "black" and *felinus* meaning "of or belonging to a cat".

BLACK PEOPLE

Negrophobia (SP) — From Latin *nigrum* meaning "black". A less preferred term is Colourphobia.[8]

BLACK UNDERWEAR

Melcrytovestimentaphobia (TP) — From Greek *melas* meaning "black or dark", *kryptos* meaning "hidden" and *vestimenti* meaning "clothing". The opposite of this phobia is Melcrytovestimentaphilia, the sexual attraction to black underwear.

BLEEDING

See Blood — Haematophobia.

BLIND AREAS IN THE VISUAL FIELD

Scotomaphobia (BP) — From Greek *skotos* meaning "darkness". This includes fear of a blind spot.

BLIND SPOT

See Blind Areas in the Visual Field — Scotomaphobia.

BLINDFOLDED (BEING BLINDFOLDED)

See Blindness (Being or Becoming Blind) — Amaurophobia.

BLINDNESS (BEING OR BECOMING BLIND)

Amaurophobia (BP) — From Greek *amaurosis* meaning "blindness or darkening". This includes fear of blindfolded (being blindfolded). The opposite of this phobia is Amaurophilia, the sexual attraction to a blind or blindfolded sexual partner.

BLOOD

Haematophobia (BP) — From Greek *haima* meaning "blood". This includes fear of bleeding, blood donating, blood injury, blood loss, blood pressure and blood transfusions. Less preferred terms are Haemaphobia and Haemophobia. The opposite of this phobia is Haematophilia, the sexual attraction to blood. In 1989, Ronald Doctor and Ada Kahn noted in *The Encyclopedia of Phobias, Fears and Anxieties* that Dr Benjamin Rush wrote of what he termed "blood phobia": "There is a native dread of the sight of blood in every human creature, implanted probably for the wise purpose of preventing our injuring or destroying ourselves, or others. Children cry oftener from seeing blood, than from the pain occasioned by falls or blows." "Blood-injury phobia" is a term sometimes used for the intense fear of blood (Haematophobia), trauma (Traumatophobia), injections (Trypanophobia) and surgery (Tomophobia).

Case: "My phobia is blood. I can't stand the sight of it. Even worse, I can't stand the taste of it. If I bite my lip and taste blood, I start to shake. When I have to get a blood test and see the blood in the tube, it makes me ill, so I look away."

★ ★ ★

SWEDISH TREATMENT FINDINGS FOR BLOOD-INJURY PHOBIA
A Swedish study of 30 patients with Blood-injury phobia found that 60 per cent of patients overcame their phobia after just one two-hour therapeutic session where "applied tension" was used. Applied tension is a technique in which the therapist teaches the patient to psychosomatically increase their blood pressure and heart rate. This prevents the possibility of the phobic patient fainting. The patients were contacted one year after the treatment and confirmed its success.

★ ★ ★

FAINTING AT THE SIGHT OF BLOOD
Approximately 15 per cent of the adult population faints when donating blood. One wonders what the fainting rate would be if those who are not willing to donate blood were included. Fainting at the sight of blood generally comes from an overactive vasovagal response. This is an evolutionary fear reflex. This response slows down the heart

rate and lowers blood pressure, causing blood to drain to the legs. Less oxygen-rich blood gets to the brain, producing light-headedness, dizziness and faintness, which sometimes results in syncope (fainting).[9]

* * *

BLOOD DONATING

See **Blood** — Haematophobia.

BLOOD INJURY

See **Blood** — Haematophobia.

BLOOD LOSS

See **Blood** — Haematophobia.

BLOOD PRESSURE

See **Blood** — Haematophobia.

BLOOD TRANSFUSIONS

See **Blood** — Haematophobia.

BLUE (COLOUR OR WORD)

Cyanophobia (NP) — From Greek *kyanos* meaning "blue or dark blue substance".

BLUSHING

Erythrophobia (BP) — From Greek *erythros* meaning "blushing or red". Less preferred terms are Ereuthophobia, Ereuthrophobia, Erthyrophobia and Erytophobia.

BOATS

See **Ships** — Nautophobia.

BODY DEFECTS

See **Deformity** — Dysmorphophobia.

BODY DIRT (ANOTHER'S)

Mysophobia (BP) — From Greek *mysos* meaning "unclean or defilement". A less preferred term is Dysomophobia. The opposite of this phobia is Mysophilia, the sexual attraction to strong body odour or dirt of a sexual partner.

BODY DIRT (ONE'S OWN)

Automysophobia (BP) — From Greek *auto* meaning "self" and *mysos* meaning "unclean or defilement". A less preferred term is Autodysomophobia. The opposite of this phobia is Automysophilia, the sexual attraction to one's own strong body odour or dirt.[10]

BODY FLUIDS

Hygrophobia (NP) — From Greek *hygro* meaning "moist". This includes fear of body secretions and sweating. The opposite of this phobia is Hygrophilia, the sexual attraction to body fluids.

BODY IMAGE

See Deformity — Dysmorphophobia.

BODY MODIFICATIONS

Stigmatophobia (BP) — From Greek *stigma* meaning "mark with a puncture". The opposite of this phobia is Stigmatophilia, the sexual attraction to body modifications or body modifications of a sexual partner.

BODY MOVEMENT

Ambulaphobia (BP) — From Latin *ambulare* meaning "to move".

BODY ODOUR (ANOTHER'S)

Dysomophobia (BP) — From Greek *dys* meaning "bad or abnormal" and *soma* meaning "body". This includes fear of odour (another's).

BODY ODOUR (ONE'S OWN)

Autodysomophobia (BP) — From Greek *auto* meaning "self", *dys* meaning "bad or abnormal" and *soma* meaning "body". This includes fear of odour (one's own). Less preferred terms are Autodysosmophobia, Automysophobia, Bromidrophobia, Bromidrosiphobia, Olfactophobia, Osmophobia and Osphresiophobia.

BODY ODOUR EMBARRASSMENT (ANOTHER'S)

Bromidrosiphobia (SP) — From Greek *bromos* meaning "stench" and *drosos* meaning "moisture". This includes fear of odour embarrassment (another's). Less preferred terms are Autodysomophobia, Autodysosmophobia, Automysophobia, Bromidrophobia, Olfactophobia, Osmophobia and Osphresiophobia.

BODY ODOUR EMBARRASSMENT (ONE'S OWN)

Osphresiophobia (SP) — From Greek *osphresio* meaning "to smell". This includes fear of odour embarrassment (one's own). Less preferred terms are Autodysomophobia, Autodysosmophobia, Automysophobia, Bromidrophobia, Olfactophobia, Osmophobia and Osphresiophobia.

BODY SECRETIONS

See Body Fluids — Hygrophobia.

BOGEYMAN

Bogeyphobia (CP) — From Scottish *bogie* meaning "spectre or goblin". Less preferred terms are Bgeyphobia, Bogiephobia and Bogyphobia. This imaginary creature takes many forms and exists in many cultures. It is most often used by parents to frighten children into obedience. For example, in Greece, the *baboulas* lives under a child's bed and is used to keep the child in bed. Some individuals keep their fear of the Bogeyman past childhood and throughout life. If you are a Bogeyphobe, you share this with US actress, singer and songwriter Jennifer Love Hewitt. Hewitt is supposedly terrified in particular by "monsters under the bed".[11]

BOLSHEVISM

Bolshephobia (CP) — From Greek *bola* meaning "throw or overthrow". It can refer to fear of Bolshevik doctrine, gatherings, people, rituals or anything else Bolshevik. A less preferred term is Boshephobia. The Bolsheviks overthrew the Russian government in 1917 and the Cold War is long since over. Nevertheless, Bolshephobia remains for some, but is certainly less common today. An example of the extent to which some Bolshephobes would go to protect themselves is US character actor Eugene Pallette, who is perhaps best known for his portrayal of Friar Tuck in *The Adventures of Robin Hood* (1938). Pallette in his later years was so terrified of Bolshevism that he barricaded himself in a well-stocked rural property in Oregon. He was convinced that the Russians would soon attack.[12]

BOOKS

Bibliophobia (TP) — From Greek *biblion* meaning "book".[13]

BOOTS

Altocalciphobia (TP) — From Latin *altus* meaning "high" and *calx* meaning "heel". This includes fear of high-heeled shoes. The opposite of this phobia is Altocalciphilia, the sexual attraction to boots or shoes with high heels.

BOREDOM

Forarephobia (NP) — From Latin *forare* meaning "to bore or pierce". This includes fear of monotony and sameness. A less preferred term is Homophobia. Of course, there are undoubtedly more bores than those who are afraid of bores. Too bad not enough bores are afraid of themselves and would therefore stop being bores. But alas, as Voltaire said in 1738, "The secret of being a bore is to tell everything." Better to leave it at that and tell no more.

BOUND (BEING BOUND)

Merinthophobia (SP) — From Greek *merintho* meaning "string". This includes fear of tied up (being tied up). The opposite of this phobia is Merinthophilia, the sexual attraction to situations in which one is bound or tied up.[14]

Case: "My biggest fear is being tied up or being confined in a straight-jacket. I'm really afraid of being unable to move or breathe."

BOWEL MOVEMENTS (PAINFUL)

Defecalgesiophobia (BP) — From Latin *defaecare* meaning "to cleanse or purify" and *gesio* meaning "to guess".

BOYS

Boeiphobia (SP) — From Greek *boeiai* meaning "boy". This includes fear of young boys.

BRADYCARDIA

See Heart Disease — Cardiopathophobia.

BRAIN

Brekhmophobia (BP) — From Greek *brekhmos* meaning "front part of the skull". A less preferred term is Meningitophobia.

BRAIN DISEASE

Meningitophobia (BP) — From Greek *meningos* meaning "membrane (of the brain)". A less preferred term is Brekhmophobia.

BRASS

Aesophobia (TP) — From Latin *aes* meaning "brass".

BRASS INSTRUMENTS

See **Wind Instruments** — Aulophobia.

BREAKING RULES

See **Errors** — Hamartophobia.

BREAST MILK

See **Breast-feeding** — Lactaphobia.

BREAST-FEEDING

Lactaphobia (BP) — From Latin *lac* meaning "milk". This includes fear of breast milk and nursing mothers. The opposite of this phobia is Lactaphilia, the sexual attraction to breast milk or a sexual partner who is breast-feeding.

BREASTS

Mammaphobia (BP) — From Latin *mamma* meaning "breast". A less preferred term is Kolopophobia.

BREASTS (FEMALE)

Mammagymnophobia (BP) — From Latin *mamma* meaning "breast" and *gyne* meaning "female, feminine or woman". The opposite of this phobia is Mammagymnophilia, the sexual attraction to the female breast.

BREASTS (MALE)

Mammandrophobia (BP) — From Latin *mamma* meaning "breast" and *andro* meaning "male, masculine or man".

BREATH

Halophobia (SP) — From Latin *halitus* meaning "breath".

BRIDGES

Gephyrophobia (TP) — From Greek *gephyra* meaning "bridge". This includes fear of crossing a bridge and crossing a river. Less preferred terms are Gephydrophobia, Gephyrdrophobia and

Gephysrophobia. The noted US author John Cheever suffered from Gephyrophobia. Cheever exhibited symptoms of this, as noted by many who knew him. What must be one of the earliest accounts of Gephyrophobia comes from Hippocrates, three centuries before Christ. Hippocrates writes: "Damocles, who was with him, appeared to have dim vision and to be quite slack in body; he could not go near a precipice, or over a bridge, or beside even the shallowest ditch; and yet he could walk in the ditch itself. This came upon him over a period of time."

Case: A 65-year-old man says, "Bridges. I see myself in the middle of a bridge and the whole thing collapses. This seems foolish, I know. Bridges are not toys. They're very strong. But whenever I start to travel on one (car, bus or train) I start to worry and get nervous."[15]

BRONCHITIS

See Chronic Obstructive Pulmonary Disease — COPD-phobia.

BRONZE

Brundisiphobia (TP) — From Latin *brundisium* meaning "bronze".

BROWN (COLOUR OR WORD)

Brounphobia (NP) — From Greek *bheros* meaning "dark animal".

BUDDHISM

Buddhistophobia (CP) — From Sanskrit *buddha* meaning "awakened or enlightened". It can refer to fear of Buddhist doctrine, gatherings, people, rituals or anything else Buddhist.

BUGGED (BEING BUGGED)

See Monitored (Being Monitored) — Monitorphobia.

BUGGING

See Watching — Scopophobia.

BUGS

See **Insects** — Entomophobia.

BUILDINGS

Edificiphobia (TP) — From Latin *aedificium* meaning "building".
A less preferred term is Batophobia.

BULLETS

Ballistophobia (TP) — From Greek *ballein* meaning "to throw".
This includes fear of missiles, projectiles and thrown objects.

BULLS

Taurophobia (AP) — From Greek *tauros* meaning "a bull". A less
preferred term is Tauraphobia. If you are a Taurophobe, you share
this with US singer, songwriter and actor Lyle Lovett. According
to one report, Lovett was once mauled by a bull on his ranch
and has been terrified of bulls ever since. If so, this is certainly an
understandable reaction — and that's not bull![16]

BUMS

See **Beggars** — Mendicarephobia.

BUNGEE JUMPING

See **High Places** — Acrophobia.

BUREAUCRACY

See **Government** — Politicophobia.

BUREAUCRATS

See **Government** — Politicophobia.

BURGLARS

See **Bad People** — Scelerophobia.

BURIED ALIVE (BEING BURIED ALIVE)

Taphephobia (BP) — From Greek *taphos* meaning "a grave".
Less preferred terms are Coimetrophobia and Taphophobia. The

opposite of this phobia is Taphephilia, the sexual attraction to being buried alive. It is believed that Edgar Allan Poe, the famous US writer of mystery and the macabre, suffered from Taphephobia as well as from Claustrophobia (fear of enclosed spaces). The two phobias certainly go together!

Case: A 66-year-old woman says, "My biggest fear is being buried alive. The idea of gasping for air in the dark in a small space is awful. Can you imagine a worse way to die?"[17]

BUSES

Omnibusophobia (TP) — From Latin *omnibus* meaning "for everything or all". Buses were originally called omnibuses.

BUSHES

See Plants — Botanophobia.

BUTTERFLIES

Psychephobia (AP) — From Greek *psyche* meaning "soul or spirit" but literally meaning "butterfly". If you are a Psychephobe, you share this with Australian–US actress Nicole Kidman, English model and TV personality Nicola McLean, and a surprisingly large number of other prominent people. Kidman supposedly "developed a 'terrifying fear' of butterflies when she was a child in Australia [she was born in Hawaii and moved with her parents to Sydney when she was four]. She reveals, 'Sometimes when I would come home from school the biggest butterfly or moth you'd ever seen would be just sitting on our front gate. I would climb over the fence or crawl around to the side of the house — anything to avoid having to go through the front gate.'"[18]

BUTTOCKS

Pygophobia (BP) — From Greek *pyge* meaning "buttocks". The opposite of this phobia is Pygophilia, the sexual attraction to the buttocks of a sexual partner.

BUTTONS

Bottiaphobia (TP) — From Latin *bottia* meaning "hump or swelling". A caller to the Richard Glover programme on ABC Radio in Sydney stated that he and his son "both have a phobia of buttons". The caller said that his son still needs someone else to button up his jacket.[19]

Chapter 4
Phobias Starting with C

"The only way to get rid of my fears is to make films about them."

Alfred Hitchcock (1899–1980)

CAISSON DISEASE

See **Bends (The Bends)** — Aeroemphysemaphobia.

CAMERAS (APPEARING ON CAMERA)

Autagonistophobia (TP) — From Greek *auto* meaning "self" and *agonistes* meaning "dramatic actor". The opposite of this phobia is Autagonistophilia, the sexual attraction to cameras or sexual situations involving cameras.

CANCER

Carcinomatophobia (BP) — From Latin *carcinoma* meaning "cancer". Also meaning "cancer" is the Latin *crab*, which alludes to anything that creeps — and that is just how cancer invades the body. Less preferred terms are Cancerophobia, Carcinophobia and Carcinotophobia. Multi-phobic Woody Allen allegedly suffers from this phobia.

Case: "Here's one for your book. I'm afraid of getting cancer. I have nightmares about it. I guess I'm obsessed by a fear of cancer. Any time there is a pimple on my skin, I think it must be skin cancer. Every time I have a stomach upset, I think I have stomach cancer. When I have a headache, I think it must be brain cancer. Get the idea?"[1]

53

CANDLES

Candelaphobia (TP) — From Latin *candela* meaning "a light or torch". King Ethelred, the older brother of King Alfred the Great (849–899), was terrified of lighted candles. Johann Wolfgang von Goethe was afraid of people cleaning candles in his presence.[2]

CANED (BEING CANED IN PRIVATE)

See Beaten in Private (Being Beaten in Private) — Rhabdophobia.

CANED (BEING CANED IN PUBLIC)

See Beaten in Public (Being Beaten in Public) — Mastigophobia.

CANNABIS

Cannabiphobia (NP) — From Greek *kannabis* meaning "hemp". Cannabis refers to the drug more familiarly known as marijuana.

CAPITALISM

Capitaliphobia (CP) — From Latin *capital* meaning "stock or property". It can refer to fear of capitalist doctrine, gatherings, people, rituals or anything else capitalist.

CARBOHYDRATES

Carbohydraphobia (NP) — From Latin *carbo* meaning "coal" and *hydro* meaning "water". A less preferred term is Carbophobia.

CARNIVAL RIDES

See Carnivals — Carolevarephobia.

CARNIVALS

Carolevarephobia (TP) — From Latin *caro* meaning "flesh" and *levare* meaning "lighten or raise". This includes fear of carnival rides. English journalist and TV personality Esther Rantzen admits to being terrified of carnival rides.[3]

CARPAL TUNNEL SYNDROME

CTS-phobia (BP) — From modern terms, "CTS" is an acronym for the medical condition of carpal tunnel syndrome. CTS involves the loss of proper nerve functioning and considerable pain in the wrist.

CARRIAGES

Amaxophobia (TP) — From Greek *amaxa* meaning "wagon".[4]

CARS

Autokinetophobia (TP) — From Greek *autokineto* meaning "moves of itself". This includes fear of automobiles, motorcycles, sports utility vehicles, trucks and vehicles. Less preferred terms are Amaxophobia, Motorphobia and Ochophobia. US dancer Isadora Duncan, famous the world over for her pioneering free interpretive dance style, was terrified of cars with roofs. She felt suffocated when she had to ride in a car that was not a convertible. Her first two children (Deirdre, aged six, and Patrick, aged two) drowned along with their nurse in a car that rolled down an embankment and into the River Seine. Ironically, Duncan was strangled while riding in a convertible when her long, flowing scarf, of which she was fond, was caught in the spokes of the car's rear wheel. Others who allegedly suffered from Autokinetophobia include US comedian and member of "The Three Stooges" Shemp Howard.

Case 1: "The thing that really scares me is car accidents. I don't know anyone who has been injured in a car accident but when I drive I feel insecure. I guess I'm scared of bad drivers."

Case 2: "[I'm really afraid of] the kind of carwash where you have to sit in the car and you drive your car so your wheels go into those rails. Completely freaks me out! I never get the carwash at the gas station, even if it's free. Even if I've been driving on Highway 99 and have dead bugs and cow poo splattered all over my hood!"[5]

CARS (BEING A PASSENGER IN A CAR)

Motorphobia (TP) — From Greek *moto* meaning "to move". This includes fear of automobiles (being a passenger in an automobile), motorcycles (being a passenger on a motorcycle), sports utility vehicles (being a passenger in a sports utility vehicle), trucks (being a passenger in a truck) and vehicles (being a passenger in a vehicle).

CARS (DRIVING A CAR)

Mobilophobia (TP) — From Latin *mobilis* meaning "movable". This includes fear of automobiles (driving an automobile), driving, motorcycles (driving a motorcycle), sports utility vehicles (driving a sports utility vehicle), trucks (driving a truck) and vehicles (driving a vehicle). The opposite of this phobia is Mobilophilia, the sexual attraction to cars or trucks, especially to driving cars or trucks. If you are a Mobilophobe, you share this with Alfred Hitchcock and English actor, model and musician Robert Pattinson.

Case: "I am 27 years old. I don't have a driver's licence because I have an intense fear of driving. I had a driver's permit for one year and went out to drive five times with my husband in the car (not on the regular street, but in a business area parking lot and little streets around it). I freaked out if I even saw a car and had panic attacks. I think this is an unusual fear because I've never heard of anyone else having this kind of problem."[6]

* * *

A VIRTUAL WAY TO DRIVE DRIVING PHOBIA AWAY

Nervous drivers are being helped to overcome their driving phobias by donning Cyclops goggles that transport them to a three-dimensional virtual world. University of Manchester researchers have been testing whether volunteers with a variety of driving phobias can use virtual reality technology alongside conventional psychological therapies to help tackle their fears. The virtual reality exposure treatment (VRET) allows subjects to drive on virtual roads and confront their fears, whether they might be driving over bridges, overtaking slow-moving traffic or merging onto the motorway. According to Dr Caroline Williams, one of those involved in the research, "Phobias may develop from a real-life event but the levels of anxiety and avoidance that results become wholly disproportionate to the incident that led to the phobia and can become a major disruption to the way people lead their lives. A fear of driving, whether it has developed following a road traffic accident or for other reasons, can escalate into a situation where individuals are too scared to drive at all."[7]

* * *

CARTOONS

See Animated Characters — Animatuphobia.

CASTRATION

Castrataphobia (BP) — From Latin *castrare* meaning "to castrate or prune".

CATAMOUNTS

See Panthers — Panther-phobia.

CATARACT EXTRACTION

See Cataracts — Cataractaphobia.

CATARACTS

Cataractaphobia (BP) — From Greek *kataracta* meaning "waterfall". This includes fear of cataract extraction.

CATASTROPHE

Symphorophobia (NP) — From Greek *symphora* meaning "catastrophic disaster". This includes fear of disaster. A less preferred term is Atephobia. The opposite of this phobia is Symphorophilia, the sexual attraction to catastrophe or disaster, including involvement with death.

CATHOLICISM

Catholicophobia (CP) — From Latin *catholicus* meaning "universal". It can refer to fear of Catholic doctrine, gatherings, people, rituals or anything else Catholic.

CATS

Felinophobia (AP) — From Greek *felinus* meaning "pertaining to cats". Less preferred terms are Aclurophobia, Aelurophobia, Ailurophobia, Elurophobia, Galeophobia and Gatophobia. The opposite of this phobia is Felinophilia, the sexual attraction to cats. Shakespeare describes "some that are mad if they behold a cat" (*The Merchant of Venice*). Dr Benjamin Rush wrote of Felinophobia: "It will be unnecessary to mention instances of the prevalence of this distemper. I know several gentlemen of unquestionable courage, who have retreated a thousand times from the sight of a cat; and who have even discovered signs of fear and terror upon being confined in a room with a cat that was out of sight." It is interesting to note that several famous dictators and kings allegedly suffered from Felinophobia. These include Alexander the Great, Roman emperor Julius Caesar, Roman emperor Augustus Caesar, Mongolian leader Ghengis Khan, Henry III of France, Napoleon Bonaparte and Italian dictator Benito Mussolini. So far there has been no theory advanced as to why these leaders shared this phobia.

Case: "I can't explain it but I have always been afraid of cats. There's something about them. They're sneaky and quiet. I don't like their eyes. Not at all."[8]

CATTLE

Bovinuphobia (AP) — From Latin *bovinus* meaning "ox or cow". Among those allegedly suffering from this phobia is Lyle Lovett. Many others express this morbid fear.

Case 1: "I have for many years now been afraid of cows. Silly, I know, but when I was about 14 and fishing with a friend, I was walking along the bank to where he was when one cow in this herd started bellowing and moving towards me. I ignored it at first but as it came down the hill in my direction the rest of the herd started to follow and they gathered speed. I turned and started to walk away. Their speed increased and I started to run. Weighed down by my fishing tackle, I glanced behind me to see them still pursuing me. As I turned to look where I was going I saw the ditch too late. I fell headlong into this shallow ditch. Now expecting to be trampled by the chasing herd, I looked up to see them stopped on the edge of this ditch, which they could easily have run through, staring down at me. I quickly got to my feet and got out of the field. The cows didn't follow. To this day I hate having to go anywhere near even a single cow — a problem when I enjoy walking so much."

Case 2: "I am absolutely terrified of cows. I shake and tremble if I have the unfortunate experience of being near one or many. I cannot bear to see a picture of any because it freaks me out and my family thinks it is really funny. It is not, though, because it is ruining my life. I get a terrible feeling in my stomach and the adverts on the TV where the cows want their milk back make me shiver. The fear of cows makes me cry sometimes. I am 34 years old. Help please, if you can."

Case 3: "I want to tell you about the phobia that I have. I'm afraid of cows. Mostly dairy cows, the black and white ones. I think this originated on a scouting trip with my dad. We were walking past a field of cows when about five or six of them ran towards the fence and one actually charged it. I used to be okay with them. I remember going on a field trip to a farm where I got to actually milk a cow and that didn't bother me at all. Now I can't stand to be anywhere near them. I start to sweat and shake when one gets even remotely close to me. I've looked to see if there was a name for this phobia but I never could find one."

Case 4: "I'm 17 years old and have a HUGE fear of cows. Every time I see one I shudder. This is bad because I live in the country and there are cows everywhere! I once went to my boyfriend's house and ran from his field because I knew those cows were out to get me. My cousin also has a fear of them."[9]

CAVES

Troglophobia (NP) — From Latin *cavea* meaning "hollow place". Czech–US tennis star Martina Navratilova is allegedly terrified of caves.[10]

CELESTIAL SPACE

Astraphobia (NP) — From Greek *astra* meaning "star". Less preferred terms are Astrophobia and Siderophobia.

CELTS (THINGS CELTIC)

Celtophobia (CP) — From Latin *Celtae* meaning "the Celts".

CEMETERIES

Coimetrophobia (CP) — From Greek *koimeterion* meaning "burial place or sleeping room". This includes fear of graves, graveyards, sepulchres and tombs. Less preferred terms are Taphephobia and Taphophobia. Among the alleged sufferers from this phobia is US actress Sarah Michelle Gellar. Gellar, when the star of the TV show *Buffy the Vampire Slayer*, was so frightened of filming in real graveyards that a special "cemetery set" was built to accommodate her fear.[11]

CENSURE

See Criticism — Kritikophobia.

CENTRE ROW (SITTING IN THE CENTRE OF A ROW)

Siticentruphobia (SP) — From Latin *situs* meaning "place or position" and *centrum* meaning "centre".

CEREMONIES

Teleophobia (CP) — From Greek *telos* meaning "end". This includes fear of award ceremonies, graduations, religious ceremonies, retirement ceremonies and weddings.

CHALLENGE TO OFFICIAL DOCTRINE, STORY, ORTHODOXY OR THEORY

See Heresy — Hereiophobia.

CHANGE

See New (Anything New) — Neophobia.

CHAOS

Chaosophobia (CP) — From Greek *khaos* meaning "an abyss or a gaping, vast, empty opening".

CHARGED FOR SEX (BEING CHARGED FOR SEX)

See Robbed (Being Robbed) — Chrematistophobia.

CHARGING FOR SEX

See Robbing — Harpaxophobia.

CHASED (BEING CHASED)

Phygephobia (SP) — From Greek *phyge* meaning "flight (as in a fugitive fleeing)". The opposite of this phobia is Phygephilia, the sexual attraction to being chased.

CHEER

See Happiness (Being Happy) — Cherophobia.

CHEESE

Turophobia (TP) — From Greek *turos* meaning "cheese". The famous 18th century surgeon Antoine Le Camus described a fellow who had such an aversion to cheese, as well as milk, "that he couldn't even smell or see it without falling in a faint".[12]

CHEMICALS

Chemophobia (NP) — From Greek *khemeioa* meaning "chemicals".

CHEMOTHERAPY

Chemotherapiephobia (TP) — From Greek *khemeioa* meaning "chemicals" and *therapie* meaning "therapy". The famous German biochemist Paul Ehrlich (1854–1915) coined "chemotherapy" in 1907.

CHEST PAINS

See Narrowness — Anginophobia.

CHEWING GUM

Mastichegummiphobia (TP) — From Latin *mastiche* meaning "masticate or chew" and *gummi* meaning "gum". US actress and TV personality Oprah Winfrey is supposedly terrified of chewing gum. According to one report, "Oprah's grandmother used to stick her chewing gum on her own furniture. It grossed out O[prah] so much that she cannot stand chewing gum to this day."

Case: "I just wanted to inform you of my phobia of chewing gum. Why does the phobia exist, you ask? Well, it began after having several dreams in which my teeth fell out after chewing gum. It's weird but every time I dream of chewing gum, the gum sticks to my teeth, and then when I try to unstick the gum, it pulls the teeth out. Because of these frequent dreams I fear chewing gum."[13]

CHICKENS

Alektorophobia (AP) — From Greek *alektor* meaning "rooster". The French surgeon Antoine Le Camus wrote that the Roman emperor Germanicus Caesar could not stand the sight or sound of a rooster. Among those suffering from this phobia is US model and actress Shannon Elizabeth.[14]

CHILDBIRTH

Tocophobia (BP) — From Greek *tokos* meaning "childbirth". Less preferred terms are Lockiophobia, Maieusiophobia and Parturiphobia.

CHILDREN

Paedophobia (SP) — From Greek *paidos* meaning "child". Less preferred terms are Paediophobia, Paediphobia, Pediophobia, Pediphobia and Pedophobia. It has been said that Woody Allen suffers from a fear of children. The opposite of this phobia is Paedophilia, the sexual attraction to children.[15]

CHINA (THINGS CHINESE)

Sinophobia (CP) — From Greek *Sinai* meaning "Chinese". A less preferred term is Chinophobia.

CHINS

Geniophobia (BP) — From Greek *genio* meaning "chin or jawbone".

CHIVES

See Garlic — Alliumphobia.

CHLAMYDIA

Chlamydia-phobia (BP) — From Greek *khlamys* meaning "mantle". Chlamydia is a sexually transmitted disease.

CHOKING (BEING CHOKED)

Pnigophobia (BP) — From Greek *pnygyros* meaning "choking". This includes fear of gagging, hyperventilating, strangling and suffocating. Less preferred terms are Anginophobia and Pnigerophobia.

Case: A 72-year-old woman says, "I once choked on a piece of meat and almost passed out. Fortunately, it went down my throat. Since then I *always* eat slowly and chew my food well. I also cut up all of the food on my plate into very tiny morsels before I start eating. This way I am less likely to choke. I guess this works, as I'm still here."

CHOLERA

Choleraphobia (BP) — From Latin *chole* meaning "bile". Cholera is a medical condition characterised by gastroenteritis-like symptoms that are caused by enterotoxin-producing strains of the bacterium *Vibrio cholera*. Less preferred terms are Cholerophobia and Choloreaphobia.

CHOLESTEROL

Cholesterophobia (NP) — From Greek *khole* meaning "bile" and *steros* meaning "solid and stiff".

CHOPSTICKS

Consecotaleophobia (TP) — From Latin *consecutus* meaning "following closely together".

CHRISTIANITY

Christophobia (CP) — From Latin *Christianus* meaning "followers of Christ". It can refer to fear of Christian doctrine, gatherings, people, rituals or anything else Christian.

CHRONIC FATIGUE SYNDROME

CFS-phobia (BP) — From modern terms, "CFS" is an acronym for the medical condition of chronic fatigue syndrome.

CHRONIC OBSTRUCTIVE PULMONARY DISEASE

COPD-phobia (BP) — From modern terms, "COPD" is an acronym for the medical condition of chronic obstructive pulmonary disease. This includes fear of asthma, bronchitis, emphysema and lung disease.

CHRONIC PAIN

Chronospoinephobia (BP) — From Greek *khronos* meaning "time" and *poine* meaning "pain or punishment".

CHURCHES

Ecclesiophobia (CP) — From Greek *ekklesia* meaning "the church". John Bunyan, the English minister and author of *The Pilgrim's Progress* (1678), suffered from Ecclesiophobia. He was terrified of both church steeples and the bell housed within them. Bunyan demonstrated the often-observed tendency for an untreated phobia to spread. At first he was afraid that the bell would toll, then that it might fall, and then that the bell, along with the steeple, might fall. Bunyan himself describes classic phobic symptoms: "How if the steeple itself should fall? And this thought, it may fall from aught I know, when I stood and looked on, did continually so shake my mind, that I durst not stand at the steeple door any longer, but was forced to flee, for fear the steeple would fall upon my head."[16]

CIGAR SMOKING

See Smoking — Smykheinophobia.

CIGARETTE SMOKING

See Smoking — Smykheinophobia.

CIGARETTES

See Smoking — Smykheinophobia.

CIGARS

See Smoking — Smykheinophobia.

CLASSROOMS

See Theatres — Theatrophobia.

CLAWED (BEING CLAWED)

See Scratched (Being Scratched) — Amychophobia.

CLAWS

See Scratched (Being Scratched) — Amychophobia.

CLEANLINESS

Arhypophobia (NP) — From Greek *a* meaning "not or against" and *rhyparos* meaning "dirty".

CLEAVAGE

See Fissures — Fissuraphobia.

CLIFFS

Cremnophobia (NP) — From Greek *kremannynai* meaning "to hang". This includes fear of precipices and steep slopes.

CLIMATE

Climatephobia (NP) — From Greek *klima* meaning "region or zone".

CLIMBING

Ascendarephobia (BP) — From Latin *ascendare* meaning "to ascend".

CLIMBING RAMPS

See Stairs — Climacophobia.

CLIMBING STAIRS

See Stairs — Climacophobia.

CLOCKS

Chronomentrophobia (TP) — From Greek *khronos* meaning "time" and *metron* meaning "measure". A less preferred term is Chronophobia.

CLOSED SPACES

See Enclosed Spaces — Claustrophobia.

CLOSETS (BEING IN A CLOSET)

See Enclosed Spaces — Claustrophobia.

CLOTHING

Vestiphobia (TP) — From Greek *vest* meaning "clothes". A less preferred term is Vestiophobia. US actor and director Tommy Lee Jones allegedly suffers from a phobia of clothing labels. US singer, songwriter, musician and actress Norah Jones claims that she is Vestiphobic as a result of social disapproval of her clothing choices.[17]

CLOUDS

Nephophobia (NP) — From Greek *nephos* meaning "cloud".

CLOWNS

Coulrophobia (SP) — From Greek *colbathristes* meaning "stilt-walker" — one of many clown talents. This includes fear of mime artists. Professor Paul Salkovskis believes that children's fears may be less to do with clowns per se and more to do with being unsettled by something as seemingly unusual as a clown. He adds, "People are typically frightened by things which are wrong in some way, wrong in a disturbingly unfamiliar way. It is almost certainly not a reaction to clowns, but we are sensitive to things which are extraordinary, particularly sensitive when we are young. My three-year-old was terrified by Peter Rabbit at a barbecue. Peter Rabbit is six inches high, not seven feet high." A caller on the Richard Glover programme on ABC Radio in Sydney stated that his "biggest fear" was clowns. Alleged sufferers from this phobia include US actor Johnny Depp, US rapper Sean "Diddy" Combs and English actor Daniel Radcliffe. As Depp put it in an interview: "[It is] something about the painted face, the fake smile, there always seems to be a darkness lurking just under the surface, a potential for real evil. I guess I am afraid of them because it's impossible, thanks to their painted-on smiles, to distinguish if they are happy or if they're about to bite your face off." Combs, according to one report, has "a strict 'No Clown Clause' in his performance contracts. He has denied this but probably because it isn't so great for his bad boy image."[18]

COAL DUST LUNG DISEASE

CDLD-phobia (BP) — From modern terms, "CDLD" is an acronym for the medical condition of coal dust lung disease. A less preferred term is (are you ready for this?) Pnumonomicroscopicsilicovolcanocovaresiophobia. The etymology of this term is from Greek *pneumonia* meaning "inflammation of the lungs", *micros* meaning "small" and *scopion* meaning "means of viewing", as well as from Latin *silicis* meaning "flint or pebble", *vulcanus* meaning "fuel of the ground (as in a volcano)" and *covare* meaning "to cover". No wonder it is less preferred. What were they thinking when they came up with this one?

COCAINE

Cocaine-phobia (NP) — From modern terms, "cocaine" is a major stimulant drug derived from a bean (cuca) of a plant native to South America.

COCKROACHES

Blattaphobia (AP) — From Latin *blatta* meaning "cockroach". US actress and singer Scarlett Johansson is reportedly terrified of cockroaches. Johansson has said, "I have been afraid of them ever since I once woke up with one crawling over my face and another was in my shoe."[19]

COITUS

Coitophobia (BP) — From Latin *coitio* meaning "coitus". This includes fear of orgasms and sexual contact involving the genitals. A less preferred term is Genophobia.

COLD (BEING COLD)

Psychrophobia (BP) — From Greek *psychros* meaning "cold". A less preferred term is Psychropophobia.

COLD (COLD THINGS)

Cheimaphobia (NP) — From Greek *cheimon* meaning "winter". Less preferred terms are Cheimatophobia, Cryophobia, Frigophobia, Pagophobia, Psychrophobia and Psychropophobia.

COLD (EXTREME COLD)

Cryophobia (NP) — From Greek *kryos* meaning "freezing cold". This includes fear of freezing.

COLLAPSING

See Weakness — Asthenophobia.

COLOURED PEOPLE (PEOPLE OF COLOUR)

Chromoanthropophobia (SP) — From Greek *khromo* meaning "colour" and *anthropos* meaning "human". Less preferred terms are Chromaphobia, Chromatophobia and Negrophobia.

COLOURS

Chromophobia (NP) — From Greek *khromo* meaning "colour". A less preferred term is Chromatophobia. Those who suffer from this phobia include Woody Allen and Billy Bob Thornton. Both find bright colours in particular difficult to live with.[20]

COMETS

Cometophobia (NP) — From Greek *kometes* meaning "long-haired" and *meteoro* meaning "lofty".

COMMITMENT

Commitmentphobia (SP) — From Latin *committere* meaning "to bring together".

COMMUNISM

Communismphobia (CP) — From Latin *communis* meaning "that which is common". It can refer to fear of Communist doctrine, gatherings, people, rituals or anything else Communist.

COMPETITION

Competeraphobia (SP) — From Latin *competere* meaning "to strive in common".

COMPLEX SCIENTIFIC TERMS

See Scientific Terms — Hellenologophobia.

COMPUTER PASSWORDS

See Passwords — Friend-or-phobia.

COMPUTER SPAM

Spamophobia (TP) — From a modern term, "spam" was originally used to refer to canned spiced ham. Now it more often refers to internet junk mail, and dates from 1993.

COMPUTERS

Computerphobia (TP) — From Latin *computare* meaning "to calculate". Less preferred terms are Cyberphobia, Cyberspace and Logizomechanophobia.

CONDOMS

Condomophobia (TP) — From Latin *cumdum* meaning "sword case". A story dating from 1706 holds that the condom was named after an English physician or earl during the time of Charles II (1630–1685). No evidence of such a person exists and condoms were already used in England for at least two centuries before Charles II was king.

CONFINED SPACES

See Enclosed Spaces — Claustrophobia.

CONFINEMENT

See Enclosed Spaces — Claustrophobia.

CONFORMITY

Normophobia (SP) — From Latin *conformare* meaning "to

fashion of the same form". This includes fear of normalcy. The opposite of this phobia is Normophilia, the sexual attraction to conformity.

CONFRONTATION

Confrontaphobia (SP) — From Latin *com* meaning "together" and *frontem* meaning "forehead", implying a face-to-face defiance.

CONGESTIVE HEART FAILURE

CHF-phobia (BP) — From modern terms, "CHF" is an acronym for the medical condition of congestive heart failure.

CONSCIOUSNESS

Consciusiophobia (BP) — From Latin *conscius* meaning "knowing or aware".

CONSTIPATION

Coprastasophobia (BP) — From Greek *kopros* meaning "faeces" and *stasis* meaning "a standstill".

CONTAGIOUS (BEING CONTAGIOUS)

Contingerephobia (BP) — From Latin *contingere* meaning "touch closely". A less preferred term is Tapinophobia.

CONTAMINATION

See Uncleanliness — Rhypophobia.

CONTAMINATION BY FAECES

Scatophobia (BP) — From Greek *skatos* meaning "dung". Less preferred terms are Molysmophobia and Mysophobia.

CONTRARINESS (BEING CONTRARY)

Ymophobia (SP) — From modern terms, "Ym" refers to the "Ym shift" in biology wherein a dimorphic fungi shifts from the yeast form in an animal body (Y) to the mould (mycelial) form in the environment (M), but only with great difficulty — quite contrary!

CONTROL

Contrarotaphobia (BP) — From Latin *contra* meaning "against" and *rota* meaning "wheel". This includes fear of losing control and out of control (being out of control).

COOKING

Mageirocophobia (BP) — From Greek *mageirikos* meaning "cooking".

CORN

Cornuphobia (NP) — From Latin *cornu* meaning "horn".

CORNERS

Cornuaphobia (NP) — From Latin *cornua* meaning "projecting point, end or horn".

CORONARY ARTERY DISEASE

CAD-phobia (BP) — From modern terms, "CAD" is an acronym for the medical condition of coronary artery disease.

CORPSES

Necrophobia (SP) — From Greek *nekros* meaning "dead body". This includes fear of dead bodies (human). The opposite of this phobia is Necrophilia, the sexual attraction to corpses.

Case: A 23-year-old man says, "My phobia is so out there. I worry that if I go to a funeral, the dead person will rise up and strangle me. If this goes in your book, please don't let anyone know it's me."

COSMIC BODIES CRASHING INTO THE EARTH

See Cosmos — Kosmophobia.

COSMIC PHENOMENA

See Cosmos — Kosmophobia.

COSMOS

Kosmophobia (NP) — From Greek *kosmos* meaning "the universe". This includes fear of cosmic bodies crashing into the earth and cosmic phenomena. Less preferred terms are Cosmophobia and Kosmikophobia.

COTTON

Xylinalinaphobia (NP) — From Greek *xylina lina* meaning "linens of wood", which is the name of cotton. English singer, songwriter, dancer and fashion designer Cheryl Cole supposedly suffers from this phobia. According to Cole, "I hate cotton wool. I went to the dentist the other day and he put it in my mouth and I felt violated for the whole day. I never use it, not for taking makeup off or anything. Even when I get my nails done they use tissues. Just the feel of it ... it squeaks. Urgh. I can't bear it."[21]

COUGARS

See Panthers — Panther-phobia.

CRABS

See Shellfish — Ostraconophobia.

CRACKS

See Fissures — Fissuraphobia.

CRAWLING ANIMALS

See Reptiles — Herpetophobia.

CREATIVITY

Creatusiphobia (BP) — From Latin *creatus* meaning "to make or produce".

CRIMES (IMAGINARY)

See Errors — Hamartophobia.

CRIMES (REAL)

See **Errors** — Hamartophobia.

CRIMINALS

Hybristophobia (SP) — From Greek *hybrizein* meaning "to commit an outrage against". This includes fear of outrageous people. The opposite of this phobia is Hybristophilia, the sexual attraction to criminals.

CRITICISM

Kritikophobia (SP) — From Greek *kritikos* meaning "able to make judgements". This includes fear of censure. Less preferred terms are Enissophobia, Enosiophobia and Rhabdophobia.

CROCODILES

See **Reptiles** — Herpetophobia.

CROSSES

See **Crucifixes** — Staurophobia.

CROSSING A BRIDGE

See **Bridges** — Gephyrophobia.

CROSSING A RIVER

See **Bridges** — Gephyrophobia.

CROSSING A STREET

See **Streets** — Dromophobia.

CROSSING A THRESHOLD

See **Thresholds** — Bathmophobia.

CROWDED PUBLIC PLACES

See **Public Places** — Agoraphobia.

CROWDED ROOMS

See **Rooms** — Koinoniphobia.

CROWDED SPACES

See Public Places — Agoraphobia.

CROWDS

Ochlophobia (SP) — From Greek *ochlos* meaning "crowd or mob". This includes fear of mobs. Less preferred terms are Agoraphobia, Demophobia, Enochlophobia and Stephanophobia. The opposite of this phobia is Ochlophilia, the sexual attraction to crowds. If you are an Ochlophobe, you share this with US actress and World War II pin-up girl Betty Grable, US actor Robert Mitchum and Woody Allen.

Case: A 27-year-old woman says, "Crowds scare me. I have a fear of being trampled. I don't even like walking against the flow of pedestrians when I'm walking one way and almost everyone else is walking in the opposite direction. My boyfriend likes going to the footy. But sitting in the stands freaks me. I feel I'll be squished by the crowd if the stadium is full. I remember watching the news when I was young and seeing soccer fans crushed against a fence. I had nightmares about that for months. I still don't like to think about that."[22]

CROWNS

Coronaphobia (CP) — From Latin *corona* meaning "crown". A less preferred term is Stephanophobia.

CRUCIFIXES

Staurophobia (CP) — From Greek *stauros* meaning "a cross". This includes fear of crosses.

CRYING

Quiritarephobia (BP) — From Latin *quiritare* meaning "to cry, wail or shriek".

CRYSTALS

Crystallophobia (NP) — From Greek *krystallos* meaning "frost". Less preferred terms are Hyalophobia, Hyelophobia and Nelophobia.

CULTS

Cultusophobia (CP) — From Latin *cultus* meaning "care, cultivation and worship".

CUMBERSOME SCIENTIFIC TERMS

See Scientific Terms — Hellenologophobia.

CURSES

Cursusophobia (CP) — From Latin *cursus* meaning "a prayer that evil should befall one". This includes fear of hexes.

CYBERSPACE

Cyberphobia (TP) — From Greek *kybernetes* meaning "helmsman". Less preferred terms are Computerphobia and Logizomechanophobia. "Cybernate" means to control industrial processes by computers. "Cyberspace" was coined by science-fiction writer William Gibson in 1982. "Cybercafe" dates from 1994.

CYCLONES

Cycloanemophobia (NP) — From Greek *kyklon* meaning "moving in a circle and whirling around" and *anemos* meaning "wind".

Chapter 5
Phobias Starting with D

"What potions have I drunk of Siren tears,
Distilled from limbecks foul as hell within,
Applying fears to hopes, and hopes to fears,
Still losing when I saw myself to win!"
William Shakespeare (1564–1616), *Sonnets*

DAMP PLACES

Topohygrophobia (NP) — From Greek *topos* meaning "place" and *hydro* meaning "wet".

DAMP THINGS

Morphohygrophobia (NP) — From Greek *morph* meaning "form" and *hydro* meaning "wet".

DAMPNESS

See Water — Hydrophobia.

DANCING

Chorophobia (SP) — From Greek *khoreia* meaning "dance". The opposite of this phobia is Chorophilia, the sexual attraction to dancing.

DARK (THE DARK)

See Darkness — Achluophobia.

DARK WOODED AREAS

See Forests at Night — Nyctohylophobia.

DARKNESS

Achluophobia (NP) — From Greek *achlys* meaning "mist". This includes fear of dark (the dark). Less preferred terms are Lygophobia, Myctophobia and Nyctophobia. The Roman emperor Augustus was not able to sit alone in the dark, according to the classic work in early psychiatry, *The Anatomy of Melancholy* (1621), by Robert Burton (1577–1640). Others allegedly afraid of darkness include Johann Wolfgang von Goethe, US author of gothic and religious novels Anne Rice, US actor Keanu Reeves, US actress, singer, dancer, producer and fashion designer Jennifer Lopez, Jennifer Love Hewitt and Robert Pattinson. Lopez was quoted as saying, "We have everything on dimmers so I kind of trick myself into the darkness. Marc [husband Marc Anthony] always turns off the lights after he comes to bed. I'm usually sleeping — or he waits till I fall asleep and then turns them off."

Case: "I'm 28. I have to sleep with a light on. I say to my partner that it's because I get nightmares. But really it's that I'm afraid of the dark. I get even more afraid if the dark room is quiet."[1]

DATING

Datusiophobia (SP) — From Latin *datus* meaning "to give, grant or offer".

DAWN

Eosophobia (NP) — From Greek *eos* meaning "dawn".

DAYDREAMING

Diesomniuphobia (BP) — From Latin *dies* meaning "day" and *somnium* meaning "dream".

DAYLIGHT

Phengophobia (NP) — From Greek *phengos* meaning "daylight". This includes fear of sunlight and sunshine. Less preferred terms are Eosophobia and Phenogophobia. French playwright Georges Feydeau, Italian director Federico Fellini and Woody Allen supposedly share an extreme fear of sunshine.[2]

DEAD BODIES (ANIMALS)

Zoonecrophobia (AP) — From Greek *zoion* meaning "animals" and *nekros* meaning "dead body".

Case: "I am severely afraid of dead animals that are stuffed or mounted on walls. I was in Yellowstone National Park and if there was a store with dead animals in it I wouldn't go in. I had to have my sister check for me to see if there were stuffed animals. One time my sister lied and told me there were dead animals in our hotel. I wouldn't go in and she forced me to go in and I burst into tears. Later I found out there were no dead animals in there."[3]

DEAD BODIES (HUMAN)

See Corpses — Necrophobia.

DEADLINES

See Time — Chronophobia.

DEAFNESS

Aklyophobia (BP) — From Greek *a* meaning "not" and *klyos* meaning "to hear". This includes fear of hearing loss.

DEATH

Thanatophobia (BP) — From Greek *thanatos* meaning "death". This includes fear of death (impending death), death of someone else and dying. Less preferred terms are Necrophobia and Thantophobia. An older expression for this phobia is *meditation mortis* meaning "thinking about death". Colombian singer, songwriter, musician, dancer and record producer Shakira admits, "I have a phobia of the subject of death. Any kind of death. Death of relationships, death of feelings, physical death including my own, but especially the death of people I love. It's something I'm working on because it's a subject that can't be avoided forever."[4]

DEATH (IMPENDING DEATH)
See **Death** — Thanatophobia.

DEATH OF SOMEONE ELSE
See **Death** — Thanatophobia.

DEATH (PRETENDED DEATH)
Pseudonecrophobia (SP) — From Greek *pseudes* meaning "false or pretend" and *necros* meaning "dead". The opposite of this phobia is Pseudonecrophilia, the sexual attraction to a sexual partner pretending to be dead.

DECAPITATION (BEING DECAPITATED)
Decapitaphobia (BP) — From Latin *caput* meaning "head" and *de* meaning "off, down, from or away". Any one of these meanings is still "Heads, you lose!"

DECAYING MATTER
Septophobia (NP) — From Greek *septi* meaning "decay or rot". A less preferred term is Seplophobia.

DECISIONS (MAKING DECISIONS)
Decidophobia (SP) — From Latin *decidere* meaning "to decide".

DECOMPRESSION SICKNESS
See **Bends (The Bends)** — Aeroemphysemaphobia.

DEEP PLACES
See **Depths** — Bathophobia.

DEER

Alkephobia (AP) — From Greek *alke* meaning "deer or elk". This includes fear of antelope, elk and moose. Woody Allen is supposedly frightened of deer.[5]

DEFEAT

See Failure — Atychiphobia.

DEFECATION

See Faeces — Coprophobia.

DEFECTS

Defectuphobia (NP) — From Greek *defectus* meaning "failure or revolt".

DEFORMED CHILDREN

Teratophobia (BP) — From Greek *teratos* meaning "monster or malformation". This includes fear of bearing a deformed child and bearing a monster. Less preferred terms are Dysmorphophobia and Teratrophobia.

DEFORMED PEOPLE

See Deformity — Dysmorphophobia.

DEFORMITY

Dysmorphophobia (BP) — From Greek *dys* meaning "bad or abnormal" and *morphe* meaning "form". This includes body defects, body image, deformed people, malformed people or ugly people. Less preferred terms are Teratophobia and Teratrophobia. The opposite of this phobia is Dysmorphophilia, the sexual attraction to a deformity or a deformed person.

Case: "This will sound strange but I find deformed people very repulsive. I don't want to ever look at one. But what is bizarre is that if I see a person with a deformity, I can't take my eyes off them and stare. I don't want to look, yet I look. When I do I get afraid. I feel my heart beating faster. I want to run but my feet are stuck in place. I don't want to stare but I do. I have nightmares of deformed people surrounding me and making me look at their deformities."

DÉJÀ VU

Paramnesiaphobia (BP) — From Greek *para* meaning "besides, near, from, against or contrary to" and *mneme* meaning "memory". Paramnesia is the clinical name for the experience of feeling sure that one has witnessed or lived through a new situation previously. *Déjà vu* is French for "already seen".

DELUSIONS

Deluderephobia (BP) — From Latin *deludere* meaning "to mock or deceive".

DEMENTIA

Dementophobia (BP) — From Latin *dementare* meaning "to be out of one's mind". Less preferred terms are Agateophobia and Maniaphobia.

DEMONS

Demonophobia (CP) — From Greek *daimon* meaning "a spirit". This includes fear of evil spirits. Less preferred terms are Daemonophobia, Demonaphobia, Demoniphobia, Demonphobia, Entheophobia and Phasmophobia.

DENTAL SURGERY

See Dentists — Dentophobia.

DENTISTS

Dentophobia (SP) — From Latin *dens* meaning "tooth". This includes fear of dental surgery. Less preferred terms are Dentaphobia and Odontophobia. The 16th US President, Abraham Lincoln, suffered from this phobia; a dentist broke off part of

Lincoln's jawbone while pulling a tooth without anaesthesia. US actor Robert De Niro supposedly avoids the dentist because he believes that he will be infected via tooth fillings.

Case: A 74-year-old man says, "I have been afraid of the dentist all my life. When I was young a trip to the dentist always meant pain, pain, pain. Now they kill pain really well but just the thought of that vibration feeling of the drill makes me break dental appointments time after time."[6]

DEPENDENCE

Soteriophobia (SP) — From Greek *soter* meaning "saviour or deliverer". *Soteria* is an ancient Greek custom of rituals and objects given to someone who has been ill or weakened in the hope that they will recover. *Sotos* is ancient Egyptian for the star we refer to by the Greek name of Sirius. Sirius was believed to be the closest star to the sun, dependent upon it, and often had a negative influence upon people.

DEPRESSANTS

See Medicines — Pharmacophobia.

DEPRESSION

Depressarephobia (BP) — From Latin *depressare* meaning "to press down".

DEPTHS

Bathophobia (NP) — From Greek *bathos* meaning "depth". This includes fear of deep places, diving, looking down and becoming dizzy, and looking down from high places. A less preferred term is Illyngophobia.

DERMATITIS

See Skin Disease — Dermatopathophobia.

DESERTED PLACES

See Alone (Being Alone) — Eremophobia.

DESERTS

Desertphobia (NP) — From Latin *desertum* meaning "a thing abandoned".

DESOLATE PLACES

See Alone (Being Alone) — Eremophobia.

DESTITUTION

See Poverty (One's Own) — Peniaphobia.

DEVIATION FROM OFFICIAL DOCTRINE, STORY, ORTHODOXY OR THEORY

See Heresy — Hereiophobia.

DEVILS

See Satan — Satanophobia.

DIABETES

Diabetophobia (BP) — From Greek *diabetes* meaning "a siphon", *dia* meaning "through" and *banein* meaning "to go". Symptoms of diabetes are great thirst and constant urination.

DIARRHOEA

Diarrhoeaphobia (BP) — From Greek *diarrhoia* meaning "a flowing through".

DIETING

Diet-phobia (BP) — From Greek *diaeta* meaning "prescribed way of life".

DINING

Deipnophobia (SP) — From Greek *deipno* meaning "dinner". This includes fear of dinner conversations, dinner parties and talking while eating.

DINNER CONVERSATIONS

See **Dining** — Deipnophobia.

DINNER PARTIES

See **Dining** — Deipnophobia.

DIRT

See **Uncleanliness** — Rhypophobia.

DISABILITY (INTELLECTUAL)

Mentalisretardephobia (BP) — From Latin *mentalis* meaning "of the mind" and *retarde* meaning "to make slow, delay, keep back or hinder".

DISABILITY (PHYSICAL)

Paraplegaphobia (BP) — From Greek *paraplegia* meaning "stroke on one side". The opposite of this phobia is Paraplegaphilia, the sexual attraction to a physically disabled sexual partner.

DISASTER

See **Catastrophe** — Symphorophobia.

DISEASE

Nosophobia (BP) — From Greek *nosos* meaning "disease". This includes fear of illness (becoming ill). Less preferred terms are Monopathophobia, Monophobia, Nosemaphobia, Panthophobia and Pathophobia. Johann Wolfgang von Goethe was supposedly terrified of disease and others whose bodies were diseased. Woody Allen allegedly suffers from this phobia.

Case: "I have a fear of disease, any disease really, but especially a disease I've never heard of before. If I hear the name of a disease, I immediately think I've got it. I know it is silly. When I first heard of prostate cancer as a teenager, I thought I must have it. I then found out it only happens to men. That did not stop me from asking if it could ever happen to a woman."[7]

DISEASE (IMAGINED DISEASE)

Pseudopathophobia (BP) — From Greek *pseudo* meaning "false" and *patho* meaning "suffering".

DISLOCATED PEOPLE

See Beggars — Mendicarephobia.

DISORDER

Ataxiophobia (CP) — From Greek *a* meaning "not" and *taxo* meaning "order". This includes fear of untidiness. Less preferred terms are Ataxiaphobia and Ataxophobia. Those who allegedly suffer from Ataxiophobia include David Beckham.[8]

DISPOSSESSED PEOPLE

See Beggars — Mendicarephobia.

DIVING

See Depths — Bathophobia.

DIVORCE

Divortiphobia (SP) — From Latin *divortium* meaning "dissolution of marriage".

DIZZINESS

Illyngophobia (BP) — From Greek *illyngo* meaning "dizziness". This includes fear of dizziness when looking down, dizziness when looking up and vertigo. Less preferred terms are Dinophobia and Vertigophobia.[9]

DIZZINESS WHEN LOOKING DOWN

See Dizziness — Illyngophobia.

DIZZINESS WHEN LOOKING UP

See Dizziness — Illyngophobia.

DOCTORS

Iatrophobia (SP) — From Greek *iatros* meaning "physician".
This includes fear of going to the doctor and iatrogenic illnesses.
Dr Benjamin Rush commented on this phobia: "This distemper is
often complicated with other diseases. It arises, in some instances,
from the dread of taking physic, or of submitting to the remedies
of bleeding and blistering. In some instances I have known it
occasioned by a desire of sick people of deceiving themselves, by
being kept in ignorance of the danger of their disorders. It might
be supposed that, 'the dread of a long bill' was one cause of the
Doctor Phobia; but this excites terror in the minds of but few
people: for whoever thinks of paying a doctor, while he can use his
money to advantage in another way! It is remarkable this Doctor
Phobia always goes off as soon as a patient is sensible of his danger.
The doctor, then, becomes an object of respect and attachment,
instead of horror."

Case: "My phobia is strange — doctors. I hate the examination,
the probing, the needles, the pain, the bad news you sometimes get
and even the smell of the doctor's surgery."[10]

DOGS

Caninophobia (AP) — From Latin *caninus* meaning "pertaining
to dogs". Less preferred terms are Cynophobia and Kynophobia.
The opposite of this phobia is Caninophilia, the sexual attraction
to dogs. If you are a Caninophobe, you share this with Irish writer
James Joyce, Shemp Howard and Woody Allen. One biographer
writes of Joyce: "Around this time [aged five] Joyce was attacked by
a dog; this resulted in a lifelong canine phobia."

Case: "My fear of dogs started when I was a little boy, maybe
four years old. I wandered into the backyard of our next-door
neighbours to find my older brother, who I thought was playing
with the boy who lived next door. The neighbours had a black dog

tied up. It was asleep and I startled it. It started to bark and jumped up on me and knocked me down. It probably did not want to hurt me and might have only wanted to play. I wasn't hurt when I was knocked down, but I was terrified. It took me 20 years before I could face up to any dog, no matter how small, especially if it was black."[11]

DOLLS

Paediophobia (TP) — From Greek *paes* meaning "child". Less preferred terms are Paediphobia, Paedophobia, Pediophobia, Pediphobia and Pedophobia. The opposite of this phobia is Paediophilia, the sexual attraction to dolls. Australian actor and producer Hugh Jackman "finds dolls that come to life creepy".[12]

DOLPHINS

See Marine Mammals — Cetusaphobia.

DOORKNOBS

Forisopomophobia (TP) — From Latin *foris* meaning "door" and *pom* meaning "knob".

DOORS

Thuraphobia (TP) — From Greek *thura* meaning "door". This includes fear of revolving doors. US actor Matthew McConaughey is supposedly terrified of revolving doors.[13]

DOUBLE VISION

Diplophobia (BP) — From Greek *diploos* meaning "double". A less preferred term is Diplopiaphobia.

DOWNSIZING

See Minimalism — Minimalphobia.

DRAINPIPES

See Drains — Suspirarephobia.

DRAINS

Suspirarephobia (TP) — From Latin *suspirare* meaning "tank at the end of the pipe". This includes fear of sliding down a drain and drainpipes.

Case 1: "I'm scared to death of drains. I'll wash dishes and bathe but I avoid drains like the plague. Whenever I get close to a drain or pool filter I freak out. I can't get my breath and my heart speeds up. I've had this since I was about three."

Case 2: "I have a fear of drains ... from little drains in the bath tub to the huge pool drain. I can't even think about touching a drain or I will freak out ... I've been afraid of them for as long as I can remember."[14]

DRAUGHTS

See Wind — Anemophobia.

DRAWN AND QUARTERED (BEING DRAWN AND QUARTERED)

Quadraphobia (SP) — From Latin *quadruplare* meaning "make fourfold".

DREAMS

Oneirophobia (BP) — From Greek *oneiros* meaning "dream". This includes fear of bad dreams and nightmares. A less preferred term is Oneirogmophobia.

DRESSED (BEING DRESSED)

See Dressing — Endytophobia.

DRESSING

Endytophobia (SP) — From Greek *endytos* meaning "dressed". This includes dressed (being dressed). The opposite of this phobia is Endytophilia, the sexual attraction to remaining dressed during lovemaking.

DRINK

Potophobia (NP) — From Latin *potare* meaning "to drink". Less preferred terms are Cibiophobia, Cibophobia, Dipsophobia, Phagophobia, Phobodipsia, Sitiophobia, Sitophobia and Turistaphobia. It may not be the act of drinking but what is drunk that is the source of fear.

DRINKING

Dipsophobia (BP) — From Greek *dipsa* meaning "thirst". Less preferred terms are Cibiophobia, Cibophobia, Phagophobia, Phobodipsia, Potophobia, Sitiophobia, Sitophobia and Turistaphobia.

DRIVING

See Cars (Driving a Car) — Mobilophobia.

DROWNING

Aquaphobia (BP) — From Latin *aqua* meaning "water". This includes fear of bathing (drowning), entering a body of water and swimming. A less preferred term is Equaphobia. Those who allegedly suffered or are suffering from this phobia are US actress Natalie Wood, US actress Michelle Pfeiffer and US model, singer and actress Carmen Electra. Wood supposedly experienced Aquaphobia her entire life. She drowned off Santa Catalina Island in California.

Case: A 22-year-old woman says that she has been afraid of drowning for as long as she can remember. "The idea of being pulled down by the water, struggling to get free, running out of air, and having water come into my mouth and lungs. I'm terrified of the very thought of this. Drowning would be the absolutely worst way to die! My boyfriend [a surf lifesaver] tells me I should get over it. But I tell him he's got to get over pushing me. I'm too afraid, I know, but it's too horrible."[15]

DROWNING (DROWNING WHILE ON A BOAT, SHIP OR VESSEL)

See Ships — Nautophobia.

DRUGS

See Medicines — Pharmacophobia.

DRUGS (MERCURIAL)

See Medicines (Mercurial) — Hydrargyrophobia.

DRUGS (NEW)

See Medicines (New Medicines) — Neopharmacophobia.

DRUGS (PRESCRIPTION)

See Medicines (Prescription) — Opiophobia.

DRUNKENNESS

See Alcohol — Methylphobia.

DRY MOUTH

Otoxerophobia (BP) — From Greek *oto* meaning "mouth" and *xeros* meaning "dry".

DRY PLACES

Topoxerophobia (NP) — From Greek *topos* meaning "place" and *xeros* meaning "dry".

DRY THROAT

Laryngoxerophobia (BP) — From Greek *laryngos* meaning "throat" and *xeros* meaning "dry". This includes fear of globus hystericus and lump in the throat (a lump in the throat).

DRYNESS

Xerophobia (NP) — From Greek *xeros* meaning "dry".

DUMMIES

See Puppets — Pupaphobia.

DUMMIES (NON-ANIMATED HUMAN DUMMIES)

See **Statues** — Statuophobia.

DUMMIES (VENTRILOQUIST DUMMIES)

See **Puppets** — Pupaphobia.

DURATION OF AN EVENT

See **Time** — Chronophobia.

DUSK

See **Night** — Nyctophobia.

DUST

Amathophobia (NP) — From Greek *amathos* meaning "dust or sand". This includes fear of sand. Less preferred terms are Amanthophobia and Koniophobia. US actor Richard Gere is alleged to be terrified of dust. According to one report, in Hollywood there "is even a joke: If you want Richard Gere not coming to your place, hang on a tablet 'Premise cleaning' and you are free from Gere."

Case: A 50-year-old woman is deathly frightened of a particular form of dust. It is the dust that forms in little balls underneath furniture. She remembers when she was a little girl playing underneath her bed. She ingested one of these balls of dust (sometimes called "dust bunnies"), began to choke, bumped her head on the underside of the bed and panicked. To this day whenever she sees a dust ball, she begins a "mini-panic".[16]

DUTCH (THE DUTCH)

Dutchphobia (CP) — From a modern term, "Dutch" is a derivation of *Deutsch* meaning "German". This includes fear of Netherlands (the Netherlands).

DUTY

See **Responsibility** — Hypengyophobia.

DWARFS

Nanosophobia (BP) — From Greek *nanos* meaning "dwarf". This includes fear of little people and midgets. The acceptable term for a dwarf is "little person".

DYING

See Death — Thanatophobia.

Chapter 6
Phobias Starting with E

"Fear is a tyrant and a despot, more terrible than the rack,
more potent than the snake."

Edgar Wallace (1875–1932), *The Clue of the Twisted Candle*

EARS (EARS OF A FEMALE)

Gynotikolobomassophobia (BP) — From Greek *gyne* meaning
"female" and *tikolobomasso* meaning "to knead the lobe". The
opposite of this phobia is Gynotikolobomassophilia, the sexual
attraction to the ears of a female sexual partner.

EARS (EARS OF A MALE)

Androtikolobomassophobia (BP) — From Greek *andro* meaning
"male" and *tikolobomasso* meaning "to knead the lobe". The
opposite of this phobia is Androtikolobomassophilia, the sexual
attraction to the ears of a male sexual partner.

EARTHQUAKES

Seismosophobia (NP) — From Greek *seismos* meaning
"earthquake". This includes fear of tidal waves and tsunami.

EATEN (BEING EATEN)

Devoraphobia (BP) — From Latin *devorare* meaning "to swallow
down or devour". A less preferred term is Phagophobia.

Case: A 34-year-old woman reports that she has been afraid of
being eaten since she was a little girl. "I remember reading a Roald
Dahl story about a mother rabbit eating her baby. I saw a nature

film of a snake eating a mouse whole. I was young at the time and I always had this fear. I thought I would be eaten by a lion, a tiger, a boa or something else. I became afraid of anything with a large mouth. This is very embarrassing but when I was with my boyfriend in high school, I didn't like when we were up close and his mouth was open. I thought he would swallow me."

EATING FOOD

See Food — Sitophobia.

EATING UNCONTROLLABLY

Phagophobia (BP) — From Greek *phagein* meaning "to eat". This includes fear of swallowing. Less preferred terms are Cibiophobia, Cibophobia, Sitiophobia and Sitophobia.

ECHOES

See Sounds — Acousticophobia.

ECZEMA

See Skin Disease — Dermatopathophobia.

EGGS

Ovophobia (NP) — From Latin *ovum* meaning "egg". Alfred Hitchcock allegedly suffered from Ovophobia.

Case: A 23-year-old woman claims that she is afraid of the sight of fried eggs on a plate. "I hate the way the yolk looks. When I look at a soft yolk I almost faint. When a person cuts into the yolk and the yellow starts to run out, I think I'm going to be cut into and will start bleeding to death. I get sick to my stomach. It makes me sick even to think about it."[1]

EIGHT (NUMBER EIGHT)

Octophobia (CP) — From Greek *octa* meaning "eight". This includes fear of the figure eight.

EJACULATION

Ejaculaphobia (BP) — From Latin *ejaculatus* meaning "to throw a dart".

ELDERLY (BEING ELDERLY)

Gerascophobia (BP) — From Greek *geras* meaning "old age". This includes fear of growing old, old (being old) and retirement. A less preferred term is Gerontophobia.

ELDERLY PEOPLE

Gerontophobia (SP) — From Greek *geron* meaning "old man". This includes fear of old people. A less preferred term is Gerascophobia. The opposite of this phobia is Gerontophilia, the sexual attraction to an old person or old people.

ELECTRICITY

Electrophobia (NP) — From Latin *electron* meaning "amber". In ancient times, amber was rubbed to generate electricity. The opposite of this phobia is Electrophilia, the sexual attraction to electricity.

ELECTROCONVULSIVE THERAPY

Electroconvulsiphobia (BP) — From Latin *electron* meaning "amber" and *convulsionem* meaning "convulsion". This includes fear of shock treatment.

ELEVATED PLACES

See High Places — Acrophobia.

ELEVATORS

Elevatuphobia (TP) — From Latin *elevatus* meaning "lift up". This includes fear of lifts. Those who allegedly suffered or are suffering from this phobia include US singer and actor Dean Martin, Woody Allen, US singer Mark McGrath and Jennifer Love Hewitt. McGrath will supposedly take the stairs unless he has to climb

40 or more flights. According to one report, Allen says, "I don't like to go into elevators. I don't go through tunnels. I like the drain in the shower to be in the corner and not in the middle."

Case: A 32-year-old woman says, "I hold my breath whenever I enter the lift [elevator] of a high-rise. The higher the building the more I'm scared. I don't like the small area, especially when it is crowded, and I'm terrified the whole thing will come crashing down. I imagine what my mangled body would look like."[2]

ELK

See **Deer** — Alkephobia.

EMBARRASSMENT

See **Social Situations** — Sociophobia.

EMPHYSEMA

See **Chronic Obstructive Pulmonary Disease** — COPD-phobia.

EMPTINESS

See **Barren Spaces** — Kenophobia.

EMPTY ROOMS

See **Barren Spaces** — Kenophobia.

EMPTY SPACES

See **Barren Spaces** — Kenophobia.

ENCLOSED (BEING ENCLOSED)

See **Enclosed Spaces** — Claustrophobia.

ENCLOSED SPACES

Claustrophobia (NP) — From Latin *claustrum* meaning "enclosed space". This includes fear of closed spaces, confined spaces, confinement, closets (being in a closet), enclosed (being enclosed), imprisonment, locked in (being locked in), locked in a confined space, locked in a house, locked up (being locked up), shut in (being shut in), small rooms (being in a small room) and small spaces (being in a small space). Less preferred terms are Cleisiophobia, Cleithrophobia and Clithrophobia. The opposite of this phobia is Claustrophilia, the sexual attraction to acts involving enclosed or small spaces. Those who allegedly suffered or are suffering from Claustrophobia include Edgar Allan Poe, Hungarian–US magician, escapologist and actor Harry Houdini, German dictator Adolf Hitler, 40th US President and actor Ronald Reagan, Dean Martin, US gridiron coach and commentator John Madden, Woody Allen, English TV travel presenter Ian Wright, US actor David Boreanaz, US actress Uma Thurman, US actress Drew Barrymore and Jennifer Love Hewitt. Martin supposedly cured himself of Claustrophobia by locking himself in the elevator of a tall building and riding up and down for hours until he was no longer panic-stricken. Thurman, according to one report, "is claustrophobic and found the experience of being buried alive in *Kill Bill 2* terrifying".

Case: A 27-year-old woman says, "When I am in a small room without windows, I feel as if the walls are closing in on me. If I look up, I'm afraid the ceiling will fall and crush me. I feel that I will suffocate. I have nightmares of being closed in. I will never live in a city. You're always closed in."[3]

END OF THE WORLD

See Apocalypse (**The Apocalypse**) — Apocalypsiphobia.

ENDLESSNESS

See Infinity — Apeirophobia.

ENEMAS

Klismaphobia (BP) — From Greek *klysma* meaning "enema". The opposite of this phobia is Klismaphilia, the sexual attraction to acts involving enemas.

ENGLAND (THINGS ENGLISH)

Anglophobia (CP) — From Latin *Anglo* meaning "Anglo-Saxons".

ENTERING A BODY OF WATER

See Drowning — Aquaphobia.

ENVY

Invidiaphobia (SP) — From Latin *invidia* meaning "envy and jealousy".

EPILEPSY

Epilepsy-phobia (BP) — From Greek *epilepsia* meaning "seizure". A less preferred term is Hylephobia. Epilepsy is a chronic neurological disorder characterised by seizures.

ERECTILE DYSFUNCTION

Medomalacuphobia (BP) — From Latin *medius* meaning "middle", *mal* meaning "bad" and *cupa* meaning "tube". This includes fear of losing an erection. A less preferred term is Mesomalacophobia.

Case: A 32-year-old man is so terrified of erectile dysfunction occurring that he has not dated since high school. "I was always afraid that if I had an erection with my girlfriend I would be unable to control myself and urinate or something else would go wrong. I was afraid I'd have an orgasm too quickly. I'm really embarrassed by this."

ERECTIONS

See Penises (Erect) — Medorthophobia.

EROTICISM

Erotophobia (CP) — From Greek *eros* meaning "sexual love". This includes fear of physical love, sexual love and sexual questions. Eros was the Greek god of love.[4]

ERRORS

Hamartophobia (SP) — From Greek *hamartanein* meaning "to go wrong or make a mistake". This includes fear of breaking rules, crimes (imaginary), crimes (real), imaginary crimes, mistakes and wrongdoings. Less preferred terms are Enissophobia, Enosiophobia, Peccatiphobia and Peccatophobia. The opposite of this phobia is Hamartophilia, the sexual attraction to a sexual partner prone to errors and mistakes, or to errors and mistakes themselves.

Case: A 33-year-old woman claims that she is a perfectionist and fears making any mistakes in anything she does that someone else can see. "I am really obsessive about checking that there are no errors. My clothes must be perfect. There must be no errors in a letter, email or text message I write. If I type a letter, I proofread it several times. If I print it out and find an error, I throw the letter away. The meals I cook for others must be cooked exactly right. If something is slightly burned I will not serve it. I throw things away if, after I buy it, I discover a flaw. I am an obsessive cleaner too. My whole life revolves around correcting mistakes, avoiding errors and hiding my flaws. My mother is this way. I was an only child. When I make a mistake I hear my mother shouting at me still. I try to be perfect but I fail. I run from my errors. I'm afraid of them."

ESCALATORS

Scalatorphobia (TP) — From Latin *scala* meaning "ladder" and *ator* meaning "up". A less preferred term is Bathmophobia.

Case 1: A 48-year-old woman says that she avoids escalators whenever she can. "When I was a little girl I had this fear of being caught in the teeth of an escalator and being slowly swallowed by it. As I struggled to free myself, people fell on top of me and crushed me. It was horrible. I still have this fear. Whenever I am on an escalator, I am very careful. I stay away from the sides and step off very quickly with a big step."

Case 2: "I have a very strong phobia of escalators, especially the ones that go down. It's a mixture of the fear of falling, of the mechanisms in the escalator jamming or breaking down, of my clothing getting caught up in the machinery, and of the other people behind me. Recently I went on a day trip to London and my friends had decided to use the Underground. Having taken one look at the escalator down to the Underground platform, I started to hyperventilate and panic. I started shaking and going white. Although I managed to eventually get to the platform by using an escalator that wasn't moving, looking down at the metal ridges in the steps made me feel dizzy and sick. I'd be interested to know if anyone else has a similar phobia."[5]

ETERNITY

Eternaliphobia (CP) — From Latin *aeternalis* meaning "of very old age".

EUROPE (THINGS EUROPEAN)

Europophobia (CP) — From Greek *Europe* meaning "the land of wide-faced people". In Greek mythology, Europa was a Phoenician princess of the city of Tyre, who was seduced by the god Zeus in the form of a white bull. Their descendants were both white and wide-faced. From Europa the continent of Europe was named.

EVALUATION (BEING EVALUATED)

See Social Situations — Sociophobia.

EVEN NUMBERS

See Numbers — Numerophobia.

EVERYTHING

Pantophobia (NP) — From Greek *pantos* meaning "everything". Less preferred terms are Pamphobia, Panphobia and Panophobia. US actor George Hamilton and English singer, songwriter and

TV personality Simon Webbe have confessed to being afraid of "everything".[6]

EVERYTHING ONE IS TOLD

See **Myths** — Mythophobia.

EVIL EYE

Ommatomalaphobia (SP) — From Latin *omma* meaning "eye" and *mal* meaning "bad".

EVIL SPIRITS

See **Demons** — Demonophobia.

EXAMINATIONS (ACADEMIC)

Examinaphobia (CP) — From Latin *examinare* meaning "to test or try". Less preferred terms are Examination-phobia and Testophobia.

EXAMINATIONS (NON-ACADEMIC)

See **Social Situations** — Sociophobia.

EXCREMENT

See **Faeces** — Coprophobia.

EXERCISE

Exercise-phobia (BP) — From Latin *exercere* meaning "keep busy, drive on".

EXHAUSTION

See **Fatigue** — Kopophobia.

EXPRESSING AN OPINION

See **Opinions** — Doxophobia.

EXPRESSING OPPOSING OPINIONS

See **Opposing Opinions** — Allodoxaphobia.

EYE PAIN

Photoalgiaphobia (BP) — From Greek *photo* meaning "light" and *algo* meaning "pain".

EYES

Oculophobia (BP) — From Latin *ocularis* meaning "of the eyes". Less preferred terms are Ommatophobia and Ommetaphobia. The opposite of this phobia is Oculophilia, the sexual attraction to the eyes of a sexual partner.

EYES (OPENING ONE'S EYES)

Optophobia (BP) — From Greek *optos* meaning "seen or visible".

Chapter 7
Phobias Starting with F

"For as children tremble and fear everything in the blind darkness, so we in the light sometimes fear what is no more to be feared than the things children in the dark hold in terror and imagine will come true."

Titus Lucretius Carus (99–55 BCE), *De Rerum Natura*

FABRICS (NON-CLOTHING)

Hyphephobia (TP) — From Greek *hyphe* meaning "web". This includes fear of non-clothing fabrics. Less preferred terms are Fabricaphobia and Textophobia. The opposite of this phobia is Hyphephilia, the sexual attraction to non-clothing fabrics.

FABRICS (SPECIFIC)

Fabricaphobia (TP) — From Latin *fabricare* meaning "to fashion and build". Less preferred terms are Hyphephobia and Textophobia.

FAECES

Coprophobia (NP) — From Greek *kopros* meaning "dung". This includes fear of excrement and defecation. Less preferred terms are Faecophobia, Rhypophobia and Scatophobia. The opposite of this phobia is Coprophilia, the sexual attraction to faeces.[1]

FAERIE TALES

See Faeries — Faeriophobia.

FAERIES

Faeriophobia (CP) — From Latin *fay* meaning "The Fates", in relation to supernatural beings. This includes fear of faerie tales.

FAILURE

Atychiphobia (SP) — From Greek *a* meaning "not" and *tyches* meaning "fortunate". This includes fear of defeat. Less preferred terms are Kakorraphiophobia, Kakorrhaphiophobia and Kakorrhaphobia.

Case: A 48-year-old man says, "I'm afraid of failure. The fear of failure is always in my mind. I'm a workaholic. I feel that if I ever let up, I'll fail. I remember my failures, especially my big failures. 'Failure' is a word not in my vocabulary, I try to tell myself. But it is. It's my biggest fear."

FAINTING

See Weakness — Asthenophobia.

FALLING

See Walking — Basiophobia.

FALLING DOWN RAMPS

See Stairs — Climacophobia.

FALLING DOWN STAIRS

See Stairs — Climacophobia.

FALSE STATEMENTS

See Myths — Mythophobia.

FANTASY ANIMALS

Pseudozoophobia (CP) — From Greek *pseudo* meaning "false or pretend" and *zoo* meaning "animal". The opposite of this phobia is Pseudozoophilia, the sexual attraction to fantasy animals.

FASCISM

Fascismphobia (CP) — From Latin *fascio* meaning "group or association". It can refer to fear of Fascist doctrine, gatherings, people, rituals or anything else Fascist.

FAT

Pinguiphobia (NP) — From Latin *pinguis* meaning "fat".

FAT (BEING FAT)

See Obesity — Obesophobia.

FATHERS

Paterophobia (SP) — From Latin *pater* meaning "father".

FATHERS-IN-LAW

Pentherophobia (SP) — From Greek *pentheros* meaning "father-in-law".

FATIGUE

Kopophobia (BP) — From Greek *kopos* meaning "fatigue". This includes fear of exhaustion. A less preferred term is Ponophobia.

FEAR (THE WORD)

See Fears — Phobophobia.

FEAR AVOIDANCE

Counterphobia (CP) — From Latin *contra* meaning "opposite, contrary to, against". This includes fear of safety from one's own phobias.

FEAR OF FEAR OF PHOBIAS

Phobophobiaphobia (CP) — From *phobos* meaning "fear, horror or aversion".

FEARS

Phobophobia (CP) — From *phobos* meaning "fear, horror or aversion". This includes fear of afraid (being afraid), fear (the word), fright, phobia (the word), phobias and terror. A less preferred term is Fearaphobia. The opposite of this phobia is Phobophilia, the sexual attraction to fears or terrors.[2]

FEATHERS

Pteronophobia (NP) — From Greek *pteron* meaning "a wing".

FEET

Podophobia (BP) — From Greek *pous* meaning "feet". A less preferred term is Briophobia. The opposite of this phobia is podophilia, the sexual attraction to feet. US actor and producer Brad Pitt allegedly suffers from Podophobia. It is reported that when filming *Troy*, Pitt "insisted on wearing leather boots instead of sandals because of his phobia of his so-called 'ugly' feet".[3]

FEMALE GENITALS

See Vaginas — Eurotophobia.

FEMALES

See Women — Gynephobia.

FEMALES IMITATING MALES

Andromimetophobia (SP) — From Greek *andro* meaning "male, masculine or man" and *mimesthai* meaning "to imitate". This includes fear of females masking gender. The opposite of this phobia is Andromimetophilia, the sexual attraction to females imitating males.

FEMALES MASKING GENDER

See Females Imitating Males — Andromimetophobia.

FENCES

Clauderephobia (TP) — From Latin *claudere* meaning "to close, block up, put an end to, enclose or confine". This includes fear of barbed wire.

FERRETS

See Weasels — Galeophobia.

FEVER

Febriphobia (BP) — From Latin *febris* meaning "fever". Less preferred terms are Fibriophobia, Fibriphobia, Fidriophobia, Fidriphobia and Pyrexiophobia.

FIGURE EIGHT

See Eight (**Number Eight**) — Octophobia.

FIGURINES

See Statues — Statuophobia.

FILTH

See Uncleanliness — Rhypophobia.

FINANCES

Chrimatophobia (TP) — From Greek *chrima* meaning "finance".

FINGER POINTING

Dactylopungerephobia (SP) — From Greek *dactylos* meaning "finger" and *pungere* meaning "to prick or pierce".

FINGERNAILS

See Nails (**Fingers or Toes**) — Onychophobia.

FINGERS

Dactylophobia (BP) — From Greek *dactylos* meaning "finger".

FIRE

Pyrophobia (NP) — From Greek *pyr* meaning "fire". A less preferred term is Arsonphobia. The opposite of this phobia is Pyrophilia, the sexual attraction to fire. It is said that Arthur Schopenhauer was so afraid of fire that he lived on the ground floor.

Case: A 41-year-old man says, "My phobia is being afraid of
fire, particularly a fire in a tall building. I once turned down a job
that would have paid me much more than I was making because
the new job would have required me to work on the 18th floor of
an office building. I'm not afraid of the height, but of a fire at that
height."[4]

FIREARMS

Hoplophobia (TP) — From Greek *hoplos* meaning "combat". This
includes fear of guns and shooting. Although he is famous for
playing spies within a world of fantasy weaponry, English actor
Roger Moore allegedly suffers from the fear of firearms.

Case: A 44-year-old man says, "I moved to Australia from the
US. In the US the concealed weapons that people carry really began
to freak me. Anyone could walk up to you and mug you — and
blow your head off if you didn't give them enough money! I'm
more relaxed in Australia, but I still sometimes get nervous when
strangers come towards me."[5]

FISH

Icthyophobia (AP) — From Greek *ichthys* meaning "fish". Among
those who suffer from this phobia are English TV personalities
Samantha and Amanda Marchant, as well as David Boreanaz. The
Marchant twins claim that they are scared of fish, "even diddy gold
ones". They say, "At supermarkets we'd run past the fish counter
screaming and refused to eat any. We couldn't even swim in the
sea or go to an aquarium — it was so embarrassing." Boreanaz
explains, "I hate fish too because they are scaly. If they come too
close I have to swim away."

Case: "I have an extreme fear of pet fish getting out of their
water, and being unable to help them while they flop around
and die. I'm not afraid of fish, just this situation. I didn't realise
how bad it was until, due to an injury, my husband couldn't

change the fish's water. The fish slid out of his hand onto the counter, flopping around, and I started to cry hysterically. I felt totally out of control and terrified. It was very weird. How about Aerokinesoichthyophobia — fish moving around in the air?"[6]

FISH TANKS

Icthyolakkophobia (TP) — From Greek *ichthys* meaning "fish" and *lakkos* meaning "pit, tank or pond".

FISSURES

Fissuraphobia (NP) — From Latin *fissura* meaning "fissure, crack, split or cleave". This includes fear of cleavage, cracks and splits.

Case: "I have a fear of things with a large number of cracks in it … like those awful posters of dry land with all the cracked ground … I get sick to my stomach. I have to look at them and I feel just gross. I almost died because there was a section of freeway that was cracked right next to my car. I was driving and freaking out, but I kept having to look at it and study it. I couldn't drive straight! I don't have any idea where this came from, but it's been a fear since I was little. If I have a scab and it cracks, it has to come off, even if I take a huge chunk of skin with it, because I can't handle the cracking."[7]

FLASHING LIGHTS

Selaphobia (NP) — From Greek *selas* meaning "flashing bright light". This includes fear of light flashes. Less preferred terms are Photoaugliaphobia, Photophobia and Phengophobia.

FLATULENCE

Flatulentiaphobia (BP) — From Latin *flatulentia* meaning "flatulence".

FLOATING

Levisiphobia (BP) — From Greek *levis* meaning "light". This includes fear of lightweight objects and things, and gravity loss. A less preferred term is Barophobia.

FLOGGED IN PRIVATE (BEING FLOGGED IN PRIVATE)

See **Beaten in Private (Being Beaten in Private)** — Rhabdophobia.

FLOGGED IN PUBLIC (BEING FLOGGED IN PUBLIC)

See **Beaten in Public (Being Beaten in Public)** — Mastigophobia.

FLOODS

Antlophobia (NP) — From Greek *antlia* meaning "moving water".

FLOWERS

Anthophobia (NP) — From Greek *anthos* meaning "a flower".
A less preferred term is Anthrophobia. Queen Elizabeth I of
England was supposedly frightened of roses.[8]

FLUTES

See **Wind Instruments** — Aulophobia.

FLYING (FLYING IN AN AIRCRAFT)

Aviophobia (TP) — From Latin *avis* meaning "a bird". This
includes fear of aeroplanes, aircraft, gliders and helicopters.
Less preferred terms are Aerophobia, Aviatophobia,
Pteromerhanophobia and Pteronophobia. Those who allegedly
suffered or are suffering from this phobia include Shemp Howard,
Ronald Reagan, US science-fiction writer Isaac Asimov, US science-
fiction writer Ray Bradbury, US actor Tony Curtis, US director
Stanley Kubrick, US comedian and actor Bob Newhart, US actress
Joanne Woodward, US singer Johnny Cash, US film and book critic
and TV personality Gene Shalit, US actress and singer Florence
Henderson, US singer Loretta Lynn, English actress and member
of the British Parliament Glenda Jackson, US daredevil stuntman
Evel Knievel, John Madden, North Korean leader Kim Jong-il,
US boxer Muhammad Ali, US singer Aretha Franklin, English
singer, musician and member of The Beatles George Harrison,
Scottish soccer star Jimmy Johnstone, US singer and actress

Cher, Hungarian–Australian–British boxer Joe Bugner, US actor
Laurence "Mr T" Tureaud, US filmmaker Barry Sonnenfeld, Billy
Bob Thornton, US comedienne and actress Whoopi Goldberg,
English musician, singer and songwriter Robert Smith, Canadian–
US actor, director and comedian Ryan Stiles, US singer Michael
Jackson, English actor Sean Bean, Danish filmmaker Lars von
Trier, US actress Sarah Jessica Parker, US actor Dean Cain, US
singer R. Kelly, US actress Jennifer Aniston, Dutch soccer star
Dennis Bergkamp, English model and designer Jade Jagger, English
socialite and writer Jemima Khan, US musician Travis Barker, US
actor Joaquin Phoenix, Irish actor Colin Farrell, English singer and
actress Kym Marsh, English singer, dancer and songwriter Sabrina
Washington, US actor Chad Michael Murray, US model, actress
and singer Kirsten Dunst, Australian model, singer and actress
Holly Valance, English soccer star Wayne Rooney, and US model
and actress Megan Fox. Aniston allegedly developed the fear of
flying after being caught in an electrical storm on a flight from
Toronto to New York City. Bean, according to one report, "didn't
like the idea of having to helicopter to certain locations during the
filming of *The Fellowship of the Ring* and after one turbulent ride
vowed never to fly to a location again. In one case he had to take a
ski lift and then hike for miles in full costume to get to the filming."
Rooney's phobia "has seen his team-mates nickname him Mr T —
after the character from the hit 1980s TV show *The A-Team* who
was famously afraid of flying".

Case: A 33-year-old man admits that he is "the ultimate white
knuckler". He adds, "I have been afraid of flying since my first
plane trip when I was 11. I worry about who's flying the plane, it
having enough fuel, it having a bomb on board, a passenger going
crazy and everything else really. I hate turbulence. When there's
turbulence I start to sweat. I'm sure the plane is going to crash. As
soon as I board a plane I say to myself, 'This is the last time'. As

soon as the plane lands I say to myself, 'Thank God!' and feel like I've dodged a bullet."[9]

* * *

FEAR OF FLYING THERAPY SUCCESS

University of Nottingham clinicians report that 84 per cent of their 38 patients with fear of flying "showed less anxiety about flying" after undergoing therapy. At one year after the therapy, 40 per cent had flown commercially and at three years after the therapy, 60 per cent had done so.[10]

* * *

A NEW VIRTUAL REALITY TECHNIQUE HELPS CONQUER FEAR OF FLYING

Researchers have concluded a study showing that a new virtual reality technique cures fear of flying (Aviophobia) after only eight therapy sessions. According to the researchers, an estimated 10 to 25 per cent of the population of all industrial nations suffers from fear of flying. This fear can cause overwhelming anxiety for those who have to travel for business, family reasons or to reach a holiday destination. Now, those with white knuckles can overcome their fear via therapy using virtual reality exposure (VRE). VRE allows a user to be an active participant within a computer-generated three-dimensional virtual world that changes in a natural way with a person's head and body movement. Findings from this study were first presented at the 108th Annual Convention of the American Psychological Association in Washington, DC.[11]

* * *

FOG

Homichlophobia (NP) — From Greek *omichle* meaning "fog or mist". This includes fear of mists and smoke. Less preferred terms are Hygrophobia, Nebulaphobia and Nebulophobia.

FOOD

Sitophobia (BP) — From Greek *sitos* meaning "food". This includes fear of eating food and foods (particular foods). Less preferred terms are Cibiophobia, Cibophobia, Phagophobia, Sitiophobia and Turistaphobia. The opposite of this phobia is Sitophilia, the sexual attraction to food. It may not be the act of eating food but the contents of what is eaten that is the fear source. English rock singer Dave McCabe is allegedly terrified of apple pies.[12]

FOODS (PARTICULAR FOODS)

See Food — Sitophobia.

FOREIGN CRIMINALS

See Foreign Thieves — Xenokleptophobia.

FOREIGN DOCTORS

Xeniaphobia (SP) — From Greek *xenos* meaning "foreign" and *iatros* meaning "physician".

FOREIGN LANGUAGES

Xenoglossophobia (CP) — From Greek *xenos* meaning "foreign" and *glossa* meaning "a tongue or language". This includes fear of languages.

FOREIGN PICKPOCKETS

See Foreign Thieves — Xenokleptophobia.

FOREIGN THIEVES

Xenokleptophobia (SP) — From Greek *xenos* meaning "foreign" and *kleptes* meaning "thief". This includes fear of foreign pickpockets and foreign criminals.

FOREIGNERS

Xenophobia (SP) — From Greek *xenos* meaning "foreign". This includes fear of strangers. A less preferred term is Zenophobia.

The opposite of this phobia is Xenophilia, the sexual attraction to foreigners or strangers.[13]

* * *

DO HUMANS HAVE AN INNATE FEAR OF FOREIGNERS AND STRANGERS?

For many decades we have known that at birth, humans show a startle reflex to the sound of a sharp, loud noise. If an infant fails to exhibit this reflex, a developmental delay is suspected. The fear of strangers develops at about six months of age and remains until about 12 months of age. Fear of unusual stimuli develops after that. These include animals, water, the dark and so on. Fear of foreigners does not develop unless it is taught or learned in some way.[14]

* * *

CAN WE BE CONDITIONED TO BE PHOBIC OF OTHER PEOPLE?

Although we have not found the phobia gene and nor are we ever likely to, we probably do have an evolved mental readiness to be fearful of certain things in our world. Does this cognitive readiness influence our relationships with other people? According to US researchers from Michigan State University, when white and black men and women volunteered in laboratory experiments that used mild electric shocks, it was found that white men and women could be conditioned to fear black men, and black men and women could be conditioned to fear white men. All other laboratory-induced fears, including any conditioned fear of women, was diminished.[15]

* * *

FORESTS

Hylophobia (NP) — From Greek *hylon* meaning "wood". This includes fear of woods (the woods). Less preferred terms are Hylephobia and Xylophobia.

FORESTS AT NIGHT

Nyctohylophobia (NP) — From Greek *nycto* meaning "night" and *hylon* meaning "wood". This includes fear of dark wooded areas and woods at night.

FORGETFULNESS

See Amnesia — Amnesiophobia.

FORGOTTEN (BEING FORGOTTEN)

Athazagoraphobia (SP) — From Greek *athaz* meaning "left behind" and *agora* meaning "marketplace". This includes fear of ignored (being ignored).

FORKS

See Pointed Objects — Aichmophobia.

FRANCE (THINGS FRENCH)

Francophobia (CP) — From Latin *Franci* meaning "the land of the Franks". Less preferred terms are Galiophobia and Gallophobia.

FREEDOM

Eleutherophobia (CP) — From Greek *eluthero* meaning "freedom".

FREEZING

See Cold (Extreme Cold) — Cryophobia.

FRIDAY THE 13TH

Paraskavedekatriaphobia (CP) — From Greek *paraskeye* meaning "Friday" and *dekatreis* meaning "the number 13". A less preferred term is Paraskevedekatriaphobia. The number 12 is considered the number of completeness (for example, 12 months of the year, 12 signs of the zodiac, 12 hours of the clock, 12 gods of Olympus, 12 tribes of Israel and 12 apostles of Christ). The number 13 upsets this completeness. The Last Supper occurring on a Friday and the Norse myth of the goddess Frigga meeting with 11 other evil goddesses plus the devil (to total 13) to plot against humans may account for the belief that if 13 are at dinner, one will die. Italian composer Gioachino Rossini suffered from this phobia and, ironically, died on 13 November 1868 — a Friday. Although the fear of Friday the 13th was and is widespread, Rossini's case is the first example of it documented among Europeans. In 2004, the Stress Management Center and Phobia Institute in Asheville, North Carolina, estimated that the phobia of Friday the 13th affects about 17 to 21 million people in the US and costs the economy $800 to $900 million in job absenteeism, travel disruption and so on.[16]

FRIDAYS

Friggaphobia (CP) — From Old Norse *Frigga*. Frigga is the goddess of married women and Friday was once known as Frigga's day. A less preferred term is Friday-phobia. The fear of Fridays goes back at least to the 14th century as it is mentioned in Chaucer's *The Canterbury Tales*. Christ was crucified on a Friday, sailors did not begin a journey on Friday, workmen did not start a new project on Friday, and many Europeans did not cut their hair or nails on Friday. The great stock-market crash of 1929 is known as "Black Friday".

FRIGHT

See Fears — Phobophobia.

FROGS

Ranidaphobia (AP) — From Latin *ranidae* meaning "frog". Less preferred terms are Batrachophobia and Bufonophobia.

Case: "I am terrified of frogs. No, really. Seeing even a picture of one makes me scream and flee. It's been this way my entire 38 years on this planet. I realise this fear is completely irrational and that the horrible creatures are harmless and possibly won't really attach themselves to my face and suck my eyeballs out, but the terror is very real to me."[17]

FROST

Pagophobia (NP) — From Greek *pago* meaning "frost". Less preferred terms are Cheimatophobia, Cryophobia, Frigophobia and Psychrophobia.

FRUSTRATION

Frustratuphobia (CP) — From Latin *frustratus* meaning "frustrate".

FUNCTIONING

See Work — Ergasiophobia.

FUR

See Animal Skins and Fur — Doraphobia.

FURRY AQUATIC ANIMALS

Lutraphobia (AP) — From Latin *lutra* meaning "furry aquatic animals". This includes fear of otters and seals.

Chapter 8
Phobias Starting with G

"Fear is that little darkroom where negatives are developed."
Anonymous

GAGGING

See Choking (Being Choked) — Pnigophobia.

GAIETY

See Happiness (Being Happy) — Cherophobia.

GAINING WEIGHT

See Obesity — Obesophobia.

GALES

See Wind — Anemophobia.

GAMBLING

Cadentemophobia (SP) — From Latin *cadentem* meaning "to fall".

GARLIC

Alliumphobia (NP) — From Latin *allium* meaning "garlic". This includes fear of chives, leeks, onions and shallots.

GASTROINTESTINAL COMPLAINTS

Gastroenterikophobia — From Greek *gaster* meaning "stomach" and *enterikos* meaning "intestinal".

Case: A 37-year-old woman says, "My phobia is stomach gas and upsets. When I first feel the pain of one I fear my stomach will explode. I watch what I eat very closely. It's not that I'm all that afraid of weight gain; it's that I'll get gastro and my stomach will explode. I used to dream about my stomach exploding just like a balloon."

GAY PEOPLE

See Homosexuality — Homophobia.

GENITAL WARTS

Genverrucaphobia (BP) — From Latin *genitalis* meaning "generation" and *verruca* meaning "swelling or wart". Genital warts is a sexually transmitted disease.

Case: A 43-year-old man claims that he is deathly afraid of any kind of blemish in the pubic region of his body. "It may be cancer, VD, herpes or a genital wart. I once had a wart on my penis. I was sure I had a genital wart since I was practising unprotected sex and was sexually active. I avoided going to the doctor for several years. Finally I did and it turned out to be a regular wart."

GENITALS (FEMALE)

See Vaginas — Eurotophobia.

GENITALS (MALE)

See Penises (Non-erect) — Phallophobia.

GERBILS

Gerbillophobia (AP) — From Latin *gerbillus* meaning "a small rodent". The opposite of this phobia is Gerbillophilia, the sexual attraction to gerbils and other small animals, usually rodents. US actress Christina Ricci reportedly suffers from Gerbillophobia.[1]

GERMANY (THINGS GERMAN)

Germanophobia (CP) — From Latin *Germanus* meaning "the land of Germans (perhaps of Celtic or Gallic origin)". Less preferred terms are Teutonophobia and Teutophobia.

GERMS

Spermophobia (AP) — From Latin *spermo* meaning "seed".
Less preferred terms are Automysophobia, Bacilliophobia,
Coprophobia, Microphobia, Mikrophobia, Misophobia,
Molysmophobia, Molysomophobia, Mysophobia, Rupophobia,
Rypophobia, Scatophobia, Spermatophobia and Verminophobia.
Those who allegedly have suffered or are suffering from this
phobia include German–US actress and singer Marlene Dietrich,
US actress Joan Crawford, US aviator, engineer, industrialist and
film producer Howard Hughes, US business magnate, socialite
and TV personality Donald Trump, Canadian actor, comedian
and TV game-show host Howie Mandell, Michael Jackson, US
actress Shannen Doherty and US actress Cameron Diaz. Dietrich
supposedly "always had a small bottle of medical spirit on call to
disinfect a toilet bowl seat with it". Hughes showed symptoms of
Spermophobia, Sociophobia and obsessive-compulsive disorder.
He went to elaborate extremes to keep free of germs. This
aversion almost certainly originated in early childhood. His overly
protective mother, Allene, was also overly concerned about
germs. *The Aviator* (2004), a film about Hughes's life, opens with
him as a young child being bathed by his mother as she lectures
him on the dangers of germs and the necessity of protecting
himself from them. Trump refuses to shake hands because of
germs. But as the editors of *Discover* magazine quip: "Does he
refuse to touch filthy money?" Mandell does not shake hands
when greeting game-show contestants. Diaz supposedly refuses
to touch doorhandles with her bare hands. Instead, she uses her
elbows to turn the knobs.

Case: A 55-year-old woman with this phobia is a nurse and
hospital administrator. Her phobia of germs extends to placing
plastic covers on the floor of her home, wiping where a glass or
cup has been placed every time a person raises it from the coffee

table, and cleaning the corners of the floor of each room with a cotton bud to make sure all the dust has been picked up.[2]

GHOSTS

See Spectres — Spectrophobia.

GIRLS

Parthenophobia (SP) — From Greek *parthenos* meaning "a virgin". This includes fear of virgins and young girls.

GLARING LIGHTS

See Lights (Glaring Lights) — Photoaugliaphobia.

GLASS

Hyelophobia (TP) — From Greek *hyalo* meaning "transparent or glass". Less preferred terms are Crystallophobia, Hyalophobia and Nelophobia. Johann Wolfgang von Goethe was supposedly terrified of people who wore eyeglasses. Although he was near-sighted from early adulthood and eventually wore a monocle, he intensely disliked those who did the same. He disliked their "hostile stare".[3]

GLASS CEILINGS

Hyeloepistegophobia (TP) — From Greek *hyalo* meaning "transparent or glass", *epi* meaning "upper" and *stegos* meaning "roof".

GLIDERS

See Flying (Flying in an Aircraft) — Aviophobia.

GLOBAL WARMING

Global Warming-phobia (NP) — From modern terms, "global warming" is the monumental climate change problem the world faces today.

GLOBALISATION

Globaphobia (CP) — From Latin *globus* meaning "globe or sphere".

GLOBUS HYSTERICUS

See Dry Throat — Laryngoxerophobia.

GLOOM

Lygophobia (CP) — From Greek *lygo* meaning "shadow". This includes fear of gloomy places.

GLOOMY PLACES

See Gloom — Lygophobia.

GOBLINS

See Spectres — Spectrophobia.

GOD OR GODS

See Religion — Theophobia.

GOING BALD

See Bald (Being or Becoming Bald) — Phalacrophobia.

GOING TO BED

See Beds — Clinophobia.

GOING TO THE DOCTOR

See Doctors — Iatrophobia.

GOLD

Aurophobia (NP) — From Greek *aurum* meaning "gold".

GONORRHOEA

Gonorrhoiaphobia (BP) — From Greek *gonorrhoia* meaning "seed or offspring". Gonorrhoea is a sexually transmitted disease.

GOOD NEWS

Euphophobia (CP) — From Greek *euphoria* meaning "bearing easily". This includes fear of hearing good news.

GOPHERS

See Moles — Soricomorphapaphobia.

GOVERNMENT

Politicophobia (SP) — From Greek *politikos* meaning "of the people". This includes fear of bureaucracy, bureaucrats, politicians and politics.

GRADUATIONS

See Ceremonies — Teleophobia.

GRAVES

See Cemeteries — Coimetrophobia.

GRAVEYARDS

See Cemeteries — Coimetrophobia.

GRAVITY

Barophobia (NP) — From Greek *baros* meaning "heavy". This includes fear of heavyweight objects and things. A less preferred term is Baraphobia.[4]

GRAVITY LOSS

See Floating — Levisiphobia.

GREAT MOLE RAT (THE GREAT MOLE RAT)

Zemmiphobia (AP) — From Greek *zemmi* meaning "small animal of the earth". The great mole rat is also sometimes known as the "naked rat" or the "great naked rat". It is believed to have an extremely strong bite for an animal of its size. One Sherlock Holmes story by Sir Arthur Conan Doyle (1859–1930) refers to the case of the giant mole rat, which was said to have been too disturbing to be described to the public. His assistant, Dr Watson, would often make references to it in other cases as well. Some were from other published stories and some were not. In Mexico and the US state of New Mexico, an obscure and mysterious mole rat is the focus of rituals and practices of underground religious cults. In the so-called Blood Eyes cult, the great mole rat is seen as a symbol of shame.

GREECE (THINGS GREEK)

Hellenophobia (CP) — From Greek *Hellos* meaning "the land of Greece". A less preferred term is Hellophobia.

GREEK TERMS

See Scientific Terms — Hellenologophobia.

GREEN (COLOUR OR WORD)

Chlorophobia (NP) — From Greek *khloros* meaning "green". A less preferred term is Grenephobia.

GROWING

See Big Objects and Things — Grossusophobia.

GROWING OLD

See Elderly (Being Elderly) — Gerascophobia.

GUILT

Nocentemophobia (CP) — From Latin *nocentem* meaning "guilty, harmful, blameworthy".

GUNS

See Firearms — Hoplophobia.

Chapter 9
Phobias Starting with H

"Fear is a noose that binds until it strangles."
Jean Toomer (1894–1967), *Cane*

HABITS

Habitusiophobia (BP) — From Latin *habitus* meaning "condition, demeanour, appearance or dress".

HAEMORRHOIDS

Haemorrhoidaephobia (BP) — From Latin *haemorrhoidae* meaning "blood flow".

HAIR

Trichophobia (BP) — From Greek *trikhos* meaning "hair-like". Less preferred terms are Chaetophobia, Trichopathophobia and Hypertrichophobia. The opposite of this phobia is Trichophilia, the sexual attraction to hair.

HAIR ("BAD" HAIR)

Hypertrichophobia (BP) — From Greek *trikhos* meaning "hair-like" and *hyper* meaning "high, beyond, excessive, above normal or over".

HAIR (EXCESSIVE HAIR)

Hirsutiphobia (BP) — From Latin *hirsutus* meaning "shaggy, long hair". US actor and producer Michael Douglas is afraid of women's hairy armpits. According to one report, Douglas was quoted as saying, "This is kind of silly, but I was just 16 and I just never thought women had hair under their arms. One summer I had this eastern European woman. It was a shock. It sticks in my mind."[1]

HAIR DISEASE

Trichopathophobia (BP) — From Greek *trikhos* meaning "hair-like" and *pathos* meaning "suffering".

HAIRCUTS

See Barbers — Barbaphobia.

HALLOWEEN

Samhainophobia (CP) — From Sanskrit *sama* meaning "season". Samhain is an ancient festival in many cultures (including the Druids), which celebrates the dead. It comes down to us today as Halloween. According to Drs Ronald Doctor, Ada Kahn and Christine Adamec, "The celebration of Halloween has its origins in fear and death".[2]

HALLUCINATIONS

Hallucinatuphobia (BP) — From Latin *hallucinates* meaning "wander (in the mind) or dream".

HANDS

Chirophobia (BP) — From Latin *chiro* meaning "hand".

HANDWRITING

Graphophobia (TP) — From Greek *graphein* meaning "to write". This includes fear of writing. A less preferred term is Epistolophobia.

HANDWRITING IN PUBLIC

Scriptophobia (SP) — From Latin *scriptura* meaning "writing". This includes fear of writing in public.

HANG-GLIDING

See **High Places** — Acrophobia.

HAPPINESS (BEING HAPPY)

Cherophobia (BP) — From Greek *chero* meaning "to be pleased". This includes fear of cheer, gaiety and mirth. Less preferred terms are Chaerophobia and Chairophobia.

HARM (BEING HARMED BY BAD PEOPLE)

See **Bad People** — Scelerophobia.

HEADACHES

Hemicraniaphobia (BP) — From Latin *hemicrania* meaning "pain in one side of the head or headache". This includes fear of migraines.

* * *

MIGRAINE HEADACHES AND PHOBIAS

Phobias are more common in migraine headache sufferers than in non-migraine headache sufferers or those who rarely have any kind of headache. This is the finding of a team of Brazilian researchers led by Dr F. Corchs of the Instituto Israelita de Ensino e Pesquisa Albert Einstein in Sao Paulo.[3]

* * *

HEARING

See **Listening** — Klyophobia.

HEARING A PARTICULAR NAME

See **Names** — Nomenatophobia.

HEARING BAD NEWS

See **Bad News** — Dysphophobia.

HEARING GOOD NEWS

See Good News — Euphophobia.

HEARING LOSS

See Deafness — Aklyophobia.

HEART

Cardiophobia (BP) — From Latin *kardia* meaning "heart". This includes fear of heart palpitations and heartbeats. A less preferred term is Cardiaphobia.

HEART ATTACK

See Heart Disease — Cardiopathophobia.

HEART DISEASE

Cardiopathophobia (BP) — From Latin *kardia* meaning "heart" and *pathos* meaning "suffering". This includes fear of angina, arrhythmia, bradycardia, heart attack, heart irregularities, high blood pressure, low blood pressure and tachycardia. Less preferred terms are Anginophobia, Cardiaphobia, Cardiophobia and Cardiapathophobia.

HEART IRREGULARITIES

See Heart Disease — Cardiopathophobia.

HEART PALPITATIONS

See Heart — Cardiophobia.

HEART SURGERY

Cardiachirurgiaphobia (BP) — From Latin *kardia* meaning "heart" and *chirurgia* meaning "work done by hand". This includes fear of post-coronary bypass surgery.

HEARTBEATS

See Heart — Cardiophobia.

HEARTBURN

Pyrosiphobia (BP) — From Greek *pyr* meaning "fire". Pyrosis is the medical term for heartburn.

HEAT

Thermophobia (NP) — From Greek *therme* meaning "heat".

HEAVEN

Uranophobia (CP) — From Greek *uranos* meaning "heaven". Less preferred terms are Ouranophobia and Siderophobia.

HEAVYWEIGHT OBJECTS AND THINGS

See Gravity — Barophobia.

HEGELIANISM

Hegelophobia (CP) — From German philosopher Georg Wilhelm Friedrich Hegel (1770–1831). It can refer to fear of Hegelian doctrine, gatherings, people, rituals or anything else Hegelian.

HEIGHT DIFFERENCES

Anasteemaphobia (NP) — From Greek *anastema* meaning "height". The opposite of this phobia is Anasteemaphilia, the sexual attraction to a great height difference in a sexual partner.

HEIGHTS

See High Places — Acrophobia.

HELICOPTERS

See Flying (Flying in an Aircraft) — Aviophobia.

HELL

Hadephobia (CP) — From Greek *Hades* meaning both the name of the Greek god of the underworld and the underworld itself. Less preferred terms are Stigiophobia and Stygiophobia.

HEPATITIS

Hepatitis-phobia (BP) — From Greek *hepatos* meaning "liver". Hepatitis is a sexually and non-sexually transmitted disease.

HEREDITY

Patriophobia (BP) — From Greek *patrios* meaning "ancestral or native".

HERESY

Hereiophobia (CP) — From Latin *heresis* meaning "school of thought of a philosophical sect", usually relating to unorthodox views. This includes fear of challenge to official doctrine, story, orthodoxy or theory, deviation from official doctrine, story, orthodoxy or theory, radicalism and unorthodoxy. A less preferred term is Heresyphobia.

HERPES SIMPLEX VIRUS

HSV-phobia (BP) — From Greek *herpes* meaning "creeping". "HSV" is an acronym for the medical condition of herpes simplex virus. HSV consists of two viruses that cause lifelong infections.

HETEROSEXUAL (BECOMING HETEROSEXUAL)

See Heterosexuality — Heterophobia.

HETEROSEXUALITY

Heterophobia (SP) — From Greek *heteros* meaning "different". This includes fear of heterosexual (becoming heterosexual), heterosexuals and opposite sex (the opposite sex). A less preferred term is Sexophobia.

HETEROSEXUALS

See Heterosexuality — Heterophobia.

HEXES

See Curses — Cursusophobia.

HIGH BLOOD PRESSURE

See Heart Disease — Cardiopathophobia.

HIGH BUILDINGS

Batophobia (TP) — From Greek *batos* meaning "height". This includes fear of passing high buildings, high objects, passing high objects, tall buildings and tall objects. Less preferred terms are Acrophobia, Altophobia, Bathophobia, Hypsiphobia, Hypsophobia and Hypsosophobia. Dean Martin suffered from an intense fear of high buildings. He preferred living in California rather than New York City because of its fewer skyscrapers.

HIGH OBJECTS

See High Buildings — Batophobia.

HIGH PLACES

Acrophobia (NP) — From Greek *akros* meaning "highest point or top". This includes fear of bungee jumping, elevated places, hang-gliding, heights, mountain climbing, mountains and skydiving. Less preferred terms are Altophobia, Bathophobia, Batophobia, Hypsiphobia, Hypsophobia, Hypsosophobia and Hysiphobia. The opposite of this phobia is Acrophilia, the sexual attraction to bungee jumping, elevated places, hang-gliding, heights, high places, mountain climbing, mountains or skydiving. Johann Wolfgang von Goethe confessed to being afraid of heights. Those who suffered or are suffering from Acrophobia include Dean Martin, US TV announcer Ed McMahon, Woody Allen, Esther Rantzen, US writer Stephen King, Irish–American actor Liam Neeson, Martina Navratilova, US singer Sheryl Crow, David Boreanaz, US actor Tobey Maguire, Sabrina Washington and Nicola McLean.

Case 1: "Heights are my fear. Being up here I generally feel safe but then when I look straight down on the platform and see how high I am it is terrifying. I have been afraid of heights since I was a little kid. It is very uncomfortable to see how high you are."

Case 2: "Heights are my greatest fear. It kind of speaks for itself. I struggle to go to the edge of the viewing platform. I can fly in a plane okay but it's the smaller heights that really bother me."[4]

HIGH-HEELED SHOES

See Boots — Altocalciphobia.

HINDUISM

Hinduistophobia (CP) — From Sanskrit *hindu* meaning "the eternal law". It can refer to fear of Hindu doctrine, gatherings, people, rituals or anything else Hindu.

HIV

See AIDS — AIDS-phobia.

HIVES

Urticariaphobia (BP) — From Latin *urtica* meaning "a nettle". Urticaria is a medical condition known more familiarly as hives.

HOBOS

See Beggars — Mendicarephobia.

HOLES

Trypophobia (NP) — From Greek *tryp* meaning "to make a hole".
Case: "Fear of putting my hands in dark holes. I've had this fear since I was very young. I put my hand inside a shoe without looking and out of the shoe crawled a swarm of earwigs. I'm not afraid of the dark, insects or holes if they're lighted — just when they're all combined! Maybe it should be called Cavuminubilaphobia since the Latin word for cavity is *cavum* and dark is *nubil*?"[5]

HOLY THINGS

Hagiophobia (CP) — From Greek *hagio* meaning "holy or saint". A less preferred term is Hierophobia.

HOME

Ecophobia (CP) — From Greek *eco* meaning "home". This includes fear of home surroundings. Less preferred terms are Domatophobia, Eicophobia, Oecophobia, Oicophobia and Oikophobia.

HOME (RETURNING HOME)

Nostophobia (CP) — From Greek *nostos* meaning "return". This includes fear of returning.

HOME SURROUNDINGS

See Home — Ecophobia.

HOMELESS PEOPLE

See Beggars — Mendicarephobia.

HOMELESSNESS

Anecophobia (CP) — From Greek *an* meaning "without" and *eco* meaning "home". Less preferred terms are Hobophobia and Mendicarephobia.

HOMOSEXUAL (BECOMING HOMOSEXUAL)

See Homosexuality — Homophobia.

HOMOSEXUALITY

Homophobia (SP) — From Greek *homos* meaning "same". This includes fear of gay people, homosexual (becoming homosexual), homosexuals, lesbians and same sex (the same sex).

HOMOSEXUALS

See Homosexuality — Homophobia.

HORSES

Equinophobia (AP) — From Latin *equus* meaning "a horse". A less preferred term is Hippophobia. The opposite of this phobia is Equinophilia, the sexual attraction to horses. US actor, director, producer and composer Clint Eastwood admits to being afraid of horses and does not like to be around them, despite his fame as an actor in Westerns. This may be due to an allergy to horses rather than a phobia. In Sigmund Freud's famous case of "Little Hans", the five-year-old patient refused to venture outside because he was terrified that a horse might bite him. Freud was determined to find out why. Hans described "black things around the horse's mouth and things in front of the eyes". This led Freud to conclude that Hans hated his father, who was represented by horses as Han's father had a black beard and wore glasses.[6]

HOSPITALS

Nosocomephobia (CP) — From Latin *noso* meaning "disease" and *komein* meaning "to tend". According to one report, US artist and filmmaker Andy Warhol suffered from this phobia.[7]

HOUSE (BEING IN A HOUSE)

Domatophobia (CP) — From Greek *domos* meaning "a house". This includes fear of property. Less preferred terms are Ecophobia, Eicophobia, Oicophobia and Oikophobia.

HOUSE PLANTS

See Plants — Botanophobia.

HUMAN BEINGS

Anthropophobia (SP) — From Greek *anthropos* meaning "human". This includes fear of human society and people. Less preferred terms are Anthrophobia, Demophobia, Phobanthropy and Sociophobia. US singer, songwriter and actress Barbra Streisand is supposedly horribly afraid of people. This is ironic since her breakthrough hit song of the 1960s was called "People".[8]

HUMAN SOCIETY

See **Human Beings** — Anthropophobia.

HUMIDITY

See **Water** — Hydrophobia.

HUMILIATION

See **Ridicule** — Catagelophobia.

HUMOUR

See **Laughter (One's Own)** — Geliophobia.

HURRICANES

See **Violent Storms** — Lilapsophobia.

HYPERTHYROIDISM

Hyperthyroid-phobia (BP) — From Greek *hyper* meaning "over" and *thyreoiedes* meaning "shield-shaped". Hyperthyroidism is a medical condition characterised by overactivity of the thyroid gland.

HYPERVENTILATING

See **Choking (Being Choked)** — Pnigophobia.

HYPNOSIS

Hypnophobia (SP) — From Greek *Hypnos* meaning the name of the Greek god of dreams. This includes fear of mesmerism. A less preferred term is Somniphobia. The opposite of this phobia is Hypnophilia, the sexual attraction to hypnosis or a hypnotised sexual partner.

HYPOGLYCAEMIA

Hypoglycaemiaphobia (BP) — From Greek *hypo* meaning "under", *glykys* meaning "sweet" and *haima* meaning "blood".

Hypoglycaemia is a medical condition characterised by hunger, shakiness, dizziness or light-headedness, loss of memory, confusion, nervousness, sweating, difficulty speaking, sleepiness, irritability, anxiety, body weakness and a tendency to have nightmares.

HYSTERECTOMY

Hysterectomophobia (BP) — From Greek *hystera* meaning "womb".

HYSTERIA

Hysterikophobia (BP) — From Greek *hysterikos* meaning "suffering in the womb".

Chapter 10
Phobias Starting with I, J & K

"What we fear comes to pass more speedily than what we hope."

Publilius Syrus (First Century BCE), *Moral Sayings*

IATROGENIC ILLNESSES

See Doctors — Iatrophobia.

ICE

See Snow — Chionophobia.

ICELAND (THINGS ICELANDIC)

Islandophobia (CP) — From Latin *insula* meaning "island". A less preferred term is Icelandphobia.

ICONS

Iconophobia (CP) — From Greek *eikon* meaning "likeness, image or portrait". This includes fear of images.

IDEAS

Ideophobia (CP) — From Greek *idea* meaning "ideal prototype". This includes fear of ideas (new ideas). Heaven help you if you are fearful of ideas and wallow in ignorance. As US literary figure Ralph Waldo Emerson (1803–1882) wrote: "Fear always springs from ignorance."

IDEAS (NEW IDEAS)

See Ideas — Ideophobia.

IGNORED (BEING IGNORED)

See Forgotten (Being Forgotten) — Athazagoraphobia.

ILLNESS (BECOMING ILL)

See Disease — Nosophobia.

IMAGES

See Icons — Iconophobia.

IMAGINARY COMPANIONS

Phantasicompaniophobia (CP) — From Latin *phantasia* meaning "imagination" and *companionem* meaning "companion". This includes fear of imaginary friends.

IMAGINARY CRIMES

See Errors — Hamartophobia.

IMAGINARY FRIENDS

See Imaginary Companions — Phantasicompaniophobia.

IMPENDING DEATH

See Death — Thanatophobia.

IMPERFECTION

Atelophobia (CP) — From Greek *a* meaning "not" and *teles* meaning "perfection or complete". This includes fear of incompleteness.

IMPOTENCE

Impotentophobia (BP) — From Latin *impotens* meaning "lacking control or powerless".

IMPRISONMENT

See Enclosed Spaces — Claustrophobia.

INANITION

See Starvation — Inanirephobia.

INCEST

Incestuphobia (SP) — From Latin *incestum* meaning "lack of chastity".

INCOMPLETENESS

See Imperfection — Atelophobia.

INCONTINENCE

See Urinary Incontinence — Incontinephobia.

INDIA (THINGS INDIAN)

Indiaphobia (CP) — From Greek *India* meaning "the region of the Indus River". A less preferred term is Katikomindicaphobia.

INDIGESTION

Indigestiophobia (BP) — From Latin *in* meaning "not" and *digestionem* meaning "to separate, divide or arrange".

INFANTILE PARALYSIS

See Polio — Poliosophobia.

INFANTS

Infantiphobia (SP) — From Latin *infantem* meaning "young child or a babe in arms". This includes fear of babies. A less preferred term is Pedophobia. The opposite of this phobia is Infantiphilia, the sexual attraction to playing the role of an infant.

INFECTION

Molysmophobia (BP) — From Greek *molysmo* meaning "infection". Less preferred terms are Misophobia, Molysomophobia and Mysophobia.

INFERTILITY

Infertiliphobia (BP) — From Latin *in* meaning "not" and *fertilis* meaning "bearing in abundance, fruitful or productive".

INFINITY

Apeirophobia (CP) — From Greek *apeiro* meaning "infinite or endless". This includes fear of endlessness.

INJECTIONS

Trypanophobia (BP) — From Greek *trypano* meaning "to bore a hole". This includes fear of syringes. Less preferred terms are Aichmophobia, Balenephobia, Balenophobia, Belonephobia, Belonophobia and Enetophobia. One study suggests that Trypanophobia affects at least 10 per cent of the population. This phobia is "a significant impediment in the health care system" resulting in some people avoiding doctors and nurses. Triggered by the pain and shock of a needle puncture, "[t]hose who inherit this reflex often learn to fear needles through successive needle exposure. Needle phobia is therefore both inherited and learned." US model and actress Eva Longoria, US singer, songwriter and actor J.C. Chasez, and Australian singer, songwriter, pianist and actress Delta Goodrem reportedly suffer from this phobia.[1]

INJURY

See Trauma — Traumatophobia.

INNOVATION

See New (Anything New) — Neophobia.

INOCULATIONS

See Vaccinations — Vaccinophobia.

INSANITY (ANOTHER'S)

Maniaphobia (SP) — From Greek *mania* meaning "mental chaos". Less preferred terms are Agateophobia, Dementophobia, Lyssophobia and Phrenophobia.

INSANITY (ONE'S OWN)

Lyssophobia (BP) — From Greek *lyssa* meaning "madness". This includes fear of madness, mania (one's own) and psychosis. Less preferred terms are Agateophobia, Dementophobia, Maniaphobia and Phrenophobia.

INSECTS

Entomophobia (AP) — From Greek *entomon* meaning "an insect". This includes fear of bugs, insects that cause itching and insects that eat wood. Less preferred terms are Acarophobia, Bug-phobia, Insectomophobia, Insectophobia and Isopterophobia. Woody Allen, English cleaning expert and TV personality Kim Woodburn, US film director, producer and screenwriter Steven Spielberg, Scottish celebrity interior designer and TV personality Justin Ryan, Nicole Kidman, English actress Lucy Benjamin, Danish model and dancer Camilla Dallerup, Scottish actor Ray Park, English celebrity chef Gino D'Acampo, English fitness trainer and TV personality Carly Zucker, and Scarlett Johansson supposedly suffer from Entomophobia.

Case: "I can't stand insects, especially the flying ones that land on your face or get into your mouth. I have a terrible fear of choking on an insect that I have swallowed. I used to believe that earwigs got their name from being able to live in your ears. I now know that isn't true. But for years I was scared that an earwig would get into my ear and hatch its eggs, and they would eat my brain. Yuck!"[2]

INSECTS THAT CAUSE ITCHING

See Insects — Entomophobia.

INSECTS THAT EAT WOOD

See Insects — Entomophobia.

INSOMNIA

Insomniaphobia (BP) — From Latin *insomnia* meaning "lack of sleep".

INTIMACY

Symbiophobia (SP) — From Greek *symbiosis* meaning "living together".

INTOXICATION

See Alcohol — Methylphobia.

IRON

Ferrumphobia (NP) — From Latin *ferrum* meaning "iron". A less preferred term is Siderophobia.

IRRATIONALITY

See Thinking (Irrational) — Aphronemophobia.

IRRITABLE BOWEL SYNDROME

IBS-phobia (BP) — From modern terms, "IBS" is an acronym for the medical condition of irritable bowel syndrome.

ISLAM

Islamophobia (CP) — From Arabic *islam* meaning "submission". It can refer to fear of Islamic doctrine, gatherings, people, rituals or anything else Islamic.

ISLANDS

Insulaphobia (NP) — From Latin *insula* meaning "island".

ISOLATION

See Alone (Being Alone) — Eremophobia.

ITALY (THINGS ITALIAN)

Italophobia (CP) — From Latin *Italia* meaning "Italy".

ITCHING

Psoraphobia (BP) — From Greek *psora* meaning "itch".

ITINERANTS

See Beggars — Mendicarephobia.

JAPAN (THINGS JAPANESE)

Japanophobia (CP) — From Japanese *Jun* meaning "sun" and *pun* meaning "place". A less preferred term is Nipponophobia.

JARGON

See Scientific Terms — Hellenologophobia.

JEALOUSY

Zelophobia (CP) — From Greek *zelotypia* meaning "jealousy". A less preferred term is Zelotypophobia. The opposite of this phobia is Zelophilia, the sexual attraction to a jealous sexual partner or involving one's own jealousy.

JET LAG

Desynchronophobia (BP) — From Latin *de* meaning "off" and *synchronus* meaning "simultaneous". Desynchronosis refers to the medical condition of disequilibrium, more familiarly known as jet lag.

JEWELLERY

Theophaniaphobia (TP) — From Greek *theophania* meaning "the manifestation or adornment of a god".

Case: "I also have a horrible phobia of jewellery to the point where I have trouble going near other people who wear it and also avoid objects that remind me of it, such as certain coins, spaghetti (the shape), some key chains."[3]

JOINT IMMOBILITY

Ankylophobia (BP) — From Greek *ankylo* meaning "stiff, crooked or unmovable".

JUDAISM

Judaeophobia (CP) — From Latin *iudaicus* meaning "pertaining to Judaism". It can refer to fear of Jewish doctrine, gatherings, people, rituals or anything else Jewish.

JUMPING

Catapedaphobia (BP) — From Greek *kata* meaning "down" and *pedo* meaning "underfoot". This includes fear of jumping from high places and jumping from low places. English singer and actress Dani Behr claims that her "big phobia is jumping out of a plane". Of course, maybe she is really afraid of falling from an aeroplane or flying itself, not jumping. Not jumping from an aeroplane unless you absolutely have to is not a phobia at all — just good sense. Skydivers think otherwise, of course.[4]

JUMPING FROM HIGH PLACES

See Jumping — Catapedaphobia.

JUMPING FROM LOW PLACES

See Jumping — Catapedaphobia.

JUSTICE

Dikephobia (CP) — From Greek *diko* meaning "justice or manner".

KIDNAPPERS

See Bad People — Scelerophobia.

KIDNEY DISEASES

Albuminurophobia (BP) — From Latin *albumino* meaning "white". Chronic kidney disease (CKD), also known as chronic renal failure, is characterised by loss of kidney function over a period of months and years.

KISSING

Philemaphobia (SP) — From Greek *philema* meaning "a kiss". A less preferred term is Philematophobia.

KNEE BENDING BACKWARDS

Gonyphobia (BP) — From Greek *gony* meaning "bent knee". Less preferred terms are Genuphobia and Kneemaphobia.

KNEES

Genuphobia (BP) — From Greek *genu* meaning "knee". Less preferred terms are Gonyphobia and Kneemaphobia.

KNIVES

See Pointed Objects — Aichmophobia.

KNOWLEDGE

Epistemophobia (CP) — From Greek *episteme* meaning "knowledge". A less preferred term is Gnosophobia.

KNOWN (THE KNOWN)

Gnosophobia (CP) — From Greek *gno* meaning "know".

Chapter 11
Phobias Starting with L

"The greatest obstacle to love is fear. It has been the source of
all defects in human behaviour throughout the ages."
Mahmoud Mohammed Taha (1909–1985), *The Second Message of Islam*

LABOUR (BEING IN LABOUR)

Parturiphobia (BP) — From Latin *parturire* meaning "to be in labour".

LAKES

Limnophobia (NP) — From Greek *limno* meaning "lake, pond, pool, marsh or swamp". This includes fear of ponds, pools, marshes and swamps.

LANDSCAPES

See Public Places — Agoraphobia.

LANGUAGES

See Foreign Languages — Xenoglossophobia.

LARGE ANIMALS

Megabiophobia (AP) — From Greek *mega* meaning the masculine form of "enormous or powerful" and *bios* meaning "life".

LARGE OBJECTS AND THINGS

Megalophobia (NP) — From Greek *megale* meaning the feminine form of "enormous or powerful". A less preferred term is Macrophobia.

LATEX

Latexophobia (TP) — From Latin *latex* meaning "liquid". This includes fear of rubber. Latex products include condoms, gloves and other items of clothing. The opposite of this phobia is Latexophilia, the sexual attraction to latex products or sexual activity involving latex products.

LAUGHTER (ANOTHER'S)

See Ridicule — Catagelophobia.

LAUGHTER (ONE'S OWN)

Geliophobia (BP) — From Greek *gelaein* meaning "to laugh". This includes humour. A less preferred term is Gelophobia.

LAVATORIES

Lavatoriphobia (TP) — From Latin *lavatorium* meaning "place for washing". This includes fear of bathrooms (public) and toilets (public). Those suffering from this phobia include Esther Rantzen and English actress, dancer, singer and songwriter Rachel Stevens. According to one report, Stevens "has a problem with locking the door to the bathroom if there's no window".[1]

LAWSUITS

See Legal Proceedings — Liticaphobia.

LAWYERS

See Legal Proceedings — Liticaphobia.

LEAD POISONING

Plumbismuphobia (BP) — From Latin *plumbum* meaning "lead". Plumbism is a medical condition also known as saturnism, Devon colic, painter's colic or, more familiarly, lead poisoning.

LEARNING

Sophophobia (BP) — From Greek *sophia* meaning "wise". This includes fear of wisdom.

LEATHER

See Animal Skins and Fur — Doraphobia.

LECTURES

See Sermons — Homilophobia.

LEEKS

See Garlic — Alliumphobia.

LEFT (THINGS TO THE LEFT)

See Left-handedness — Sinistrophobia.

LEFT BEHIND (BEING LEFT BEHIND)

See Abandonment — Abannumaphobia.

LEFT SIDE (THINGS ON THE LEFT SIDE OF ONE'S OWN BODY)

See Left-handedness — Sinistrophobia.

LEFT-HANDEDNESS

Sinistrophobia (BP) — From Latin *sinistro* meaning "left-handed".
This includes fear of the left (things to the left), left side (things
on the left side of one's own body) and left-sided objects. Less
preferred terms are Laevophobia and Levophobia.

LEFT-SIDED OBJECTS

See Left-handedness — Sinistrophobia.

LEGAL PROCEEDINGS

Liticaphobia (SP) — From Latin *litgare* meaning "to litigate". This
includes fear of lawsuits and lawyers.

LEOPARDS

Leopardosophobia (AP) — From Greek *leopardos* meaning "leopard".

LEPROSY

Leprophobia (BP) — From Greek *lepros* meaning "scabby or
scaling". Leprosy is a medical condition also known as Hansen's
disease. A less preferred term is Lepraphobia.

LESBIANS

See **Homosexuality** — Homophobia.

LETTERS

Epistolophobia (TP) — From Greek *epistole* meaning "letter or message".

LIBIDO

See **Sex** — Genophobia.

LICE

Phtheirophobia (AP) — From Greek *phtheir* meaning "a louse". A less preferred term is Pediculophobia.[2]

LIES

See **Myths** — Mythophobia.

LIFTS

See **Elevators** — Elevatuphobia.

LIGHT

Photophobia (NP) — From Greek *photo* meaning "light". Less preferred terms are Phengophobia, Photoaugliaphobia and Selaphobia.

LIGHT BULBS

Photobolbosophobia (TP) — From Greek *photo* meaning "light" and *bolbos* meaning "bulb".

LIGHT FLASHES

See **Flashing Lights** — Selaphobia.

LIGHTNING

Keraunophobia (NP) — From Greek *cerauno* meaning "bolt from the sky". Less preferred terms are Astraphobia, Astrapophobia, Astrophobia, Astropophobia, Brontophobia, Ceraunophobia,

Ceraynophobia, Selaphobia and Tonitrophobia. The Roman emperor Augustus carried a seal skin amulet at all times to protect him from his phobia of lightning.

Case: A 59-year-old woman says she has been terrified of lightning all her life. "I was playing with my friends on the school playground at recess. We didn't notice the dark clouds forming overhead. A bolt of lightning struck the playground right in front of us with the horrible sound of thunder at the same instant. It was like an explosion. It knocked me down. I cried and cried. I have been deathly scared of lightning ever since. When I hear thunder in the distance I come inside. I wait for that bolt of lightning to strike. I tried to hide my phobia from my children when they were little. I don't know if I did a very good job of this since both are scared of lightning (and thunder) too."[3]

LIGHTS (GLARING LIGHTS)

Photoaugliaphobia (NP) — From Greek *photo* meaning "light" and *auglia* meaning "glare". This includes fear of glaring lights. Less preferred terms are Phengophobia, Photophobia and Selaphobia.

LIGHTWEIGHT OBJECTS AND THINGS

See Floating — Levisiphobia.

LINGERIE

Lingeriephobia (TP) — From Latin *lineus* meaning "of linen". This includes fear of underwear. The opposite of this phobia is Lingeriephilia, the sexual attraction to lingerie or sexual activity involving lingerie.

LIONS

Leontophobia (AP) — From Greek *leon* meaning "lion".

LIQUIDS

See Water — Hydrophobia.

LISTENING

Klyophobia (BP) — From Greek *klyo* meaning "hear, be called". This includes fear of hearing.

LITTLE PEOPLE

See Dwarfs — Nanosophobia.

LIZARDS

See Reptiles — Herpetophobia.

LOBOTOMY

Lobotomophobia (BP) — From Greek *lobos* meaning "lobe (as in the brain)" and *tomos* meaning "to cut or slice". A lobotomy is a medical procedure in psychosurgery involving the cutting of connections to and from the prefrontal cortex.

LOBSTERS

See Shellfish — Ostraconophobia.

LOCKED IN (BEING LOCKED IN)

See Enclosed Spaces — Claustrophobia.

LOCKED IN A CONFINED SPACE

See Enclosed Spaces — Claustrophobia.

LOCKED IN A HOUSE

See Enclosed Spaces — Claustrophobia.

LOCKED UP (BEING LOCKED UP)

See Enclosed Spaces — Claustrophobia.

LOCKJAW

See Tetanus — Tetanophobia.

LONELINESS

See Alone (Being Alone) — Eremophobia.

LONG WAITS

See **Waiting** — Macrophobia.

LONG WORDS

See **Words (Long or Unpronounceable)** — Sesquipedalophobia.

LOOKED AT (BEING LOOKED AT)

See **Monitored (Being Monitored)** — Monitorphobia.

LOOKING

See **Watching** — Scopophobia.

LOOKING DOWN AND BECOMING DIZZY

See **Depths** — Bathophobia.

LOOKING DOWN FROM HIGH PLACES

See **Depths** — Bathophobia.

LOOKING IN A MIRROR

See **Mirrors** — Eisoptrophobia.

LOOKING RIDICULOUS

See **Ridicule** — Catagelophobia.

LOOKING UP

Anablepophobia (BP) — From Greek *anablepo* meaning "to look up". This includes fear of looking up and becoming dizzy, and looking up at high places. A less preferred term is Anablephobia.

LOOKING UP AND BECOMING DIZZY

See **Looking Up** — Anablepophobia.

LOOKING UP AT HIGH PLACES

See **Looking Up** — Anablepophobia.

LOSING A BODY PART

See **Amputations** — Apotemnophobia.

LOSING AN ERECTION

See **Erectile Dysfunction** — Medomalacuphobia.

LOSING CONTROL

See **Control** — Contrarotaphobia.

LOSING ONE'S VIRGINITY

Lysuseisodophobia (CP) — From Greek *lysus* meaning "loosening" and *eisodo* meaning "way within". Less preferred terms are Eisodophobia, Esodophobia and Primeisodophobia.

LOSING WEIGHT

See **Starvation** — Inanirephobia.

LOST (BEING LOST)

See **Alone (Being Alone)** — Eremophobia.

LOUD NOISES

See **Noises** — Ligyrophobia.

LOUD TALKING

See **Voice (Another's)** — Voxiphobia.

LOVE (BEING IN LOVE)

Philophobia (BP) — From Greek *phileein* meaning "to love". This includes fear of love (falling in love).

LOVE (FALLING IN LOVE)

See **Love (Being in Love)** — Philophobia.

LOVE (MAKING LOVE)

Agrexophobia (SP) — From Greek *agrexo* meaning "unite". The opposite of this phobia is Agrexophilia, the sexual attraction to making love while being seen or heard.

LOW BLOOD PRESSURE

See **Heart Disease** — Cardiopathophobia.

LUMP IN THE THROAT (A LUMP IN THE THROAT)

See Dry Throat — Laryngoxerophobia.

LUNG DISEASE

See Chronic Obstructive Pulmonary Disease — COPD-phobia.

LYING

See Myths — Mythophobia.

Chapter 12
Phobias Starting with M

"Am I afraid of high notes? Of course I am afraid. What sane man is not?"

Luciano Pavarotti (1935–2007)

MACHINERY

See Machines — Mechanophobia.

MACHINES

Mechanophobia (TP) — From Greek *mechane* meaning "machine". This includes fear of machinery and motors.

Case: "All my life I've been scared of large machinery. When I was a child I saw Charlie Chaplin's film *Modern Times* and was really scared when he was caught in the gears of the huge machine. I've had nightmares about that happening to me. I also don't like the loud noise big machines make. It sounds as if an animal is about to devour you!"

MADNESS

See Insanity (One's Own) — Lyssophobia.

MAGIC

Arcanophobia (CP) — From Greek *arcano* meaning "magic". A less preferred term is Wiccaphobia.

MAGIC WANDS

See Beaten in Private (Being Beaten in Private) — Rhabdophobia.

MALE GENITALS

See Penises (Non-erect) — Phallophobia.

MALES

See Men — Androphobia.

MALES IMITATING FEMALES

Gynemimetophobia (SP) — From Greek *gyne* meaning "female" and *mimesthai* meaning "to imitate". This includes fear of males masking gender. The opposite of this phobia is Gynemimetophilia, the sexual attraction to males imitating females.

MALES MASKING GENDER

See Males Imitating Females — Gynemimetophobia.

MALFORMED PEOPLE

See Deformity — Dysmorphophobia.

MANATEES

See Marine Mammals — Cetusaphobia.

MANIA (ONE'S OWN)

See Insanity (One's Own) — Lyssophobia.

MANNEQUINS

See Statues — Statuophobia.

MANY THINGS

Polyphobia (NP) — From Greek *polys* meaning "many".

MARIJUANA

See Cannabis — Cannabiphobia.

MARINE MAMMALS

Cetusaphobia (AP) — From Latin *cetus* meaning "whale". This includes fear of dolphins, manatees, porpoises and whales. US model, actress and TV personality Tyra Banks is allegedly afraid of marine animals. According to one report, Banks confronted her fear on her talk show, "but still has a little more to get over".[1]

MARIONETTES

See **Puppets** — Pupaphobia.

MARRIAGE

Gamophobia (SP) — From Greek *gamo* meaning "marriage or union". A less preferred term is Gametophobia.

MARSHES

See **Lakes** — Limnophobia.

MARXISM

Marxophobia (CP) — From German philosopher Karl Marx (1818–1883). It can refer to fear of Marxist doctrine, gatherings, people, rituals or anything else Marxist.

MASKING GENDER

Androgynophobia (SP) — From Greek *andros* meaning "male" and *gyne* meaning "female". Although fear of females imitating males is Andromimetophobia and males imitating females is Gynemimetophobia, such masking can be more complicated. The opposite of this phobia is Androgynophilia, the sexual attraction to the masking of gender in any form.

MASSAGES (BEING MASSAGED)

See **Touched (Being Touched)** — Haphephobia.

MATERIAL THINGS

See **Materialism** — Hylephobia.

MATERIALISM

Hylephobia (TP) — From Greek *hyle* meaning "substance". This includes fear of material things. Less preferred terms are Aurophobia and Hylophobia.

MATHEMATICS

See **Numbers** — Numerophobia.

MATTRESSES

See **Beds** — Clinophobia.

MEAT

Carnophobia (NP) — From Latin *carnis* meaning "meat". English model, columnist and TV personality Nikki Grahame, although not a vegetarian, has been afraid of ground meat since childhood. But this situation may have changed. According to one report, Grahame "says she's always been afraid of it [mince], until her boyfriend recently cooked it for her in spaghetti bolognese". Too bad we all cannot cook and eat the source of our phobia!

Case: "This is going to sound very strange to you, but my greatest fear is to see raw meat. I avoid thinking about it. I am a vegan. I hate walking near a butcher shop. The smell of raw meat that comes from butcher shops almost turns my stomach. I once saw cow's tongue laid out on a tray. I almost started to run away. I have fears that I will be ground up like mince."[2]

MEDICINES

Pharmacophobia (TP) — From Greek *pharmakon* meaning "a medicine or drug". This includes fear of analgesics (painkillers), antidepressants, depressants, drugs, sedatives and tranquillisers.

MEDICINES (MERCURIAL)

Hydrargyrophobia (TP) — From Greek *hydra* meaning "water" and *gyro* meaning "whirling". This includes fear of drugs (mercurial). A less preferred term is Hydragyophoia.

MEDICINES (NEW)

Neopharmacophobia (TP) — From Greek *neo* meaning "new" and *pharmakon* meaning "a medicine or drug". This includes fear of drugs (new drugs).

MEDICINES (PRESCRIPTION)

Opiophobia (TP) — From Greek *opion* meaning "opium, poppy or poppy juice". This includes fear of drugs (prescription).

MEDITATION

See Thinking (Rational) — Phronemophobia.

MEMORY (MEMORIES)

Mnemophobia (BP) — From Greek *mnemon* meaning "memory".

MEMORY LOSS

See Amnesia — Amnesiophobia.

MEN

Androphobia (SP) — From Greek *andros* meaning "male". This includes fear of males. Less preferred terms are Anthrophobia, Anthropophobia, Arrhenophobia, Arrhenphobia, Hominophobia and Masculinophobia.

Case: A 51-year-old woman says, "I have never trusted men. I have been hurt by men, as have many of my friends. I am afraid of men, especially strange men. I am physically small. I know what a large man could do to me. When I was nine I was raped by our next-door neighbour. He lured me into his backyard. He was wearing a dirty and foul-smelling T-shirt. I remember that smell to this day. I hate the smell of men. I can't stand being alone with a man, especially in close quarters."

MENOPAUSE

Menopausephobia (BP) — From Greek *men* meaning "monthly" and *pausis* meaning "a halt, stop or cessation".

MENSTRUATION

Menophobia (BP) — From Latin *menstrualis* meaning "monthly".

MENTAL ILLNESS

Phrenophobia (BP) — From Greek *phrenos* meaning "mind".

Case: A 54-year-old woman says that she is afraid of mental illness because it runs in her family. "My aunt and my sister both were institutionalised. My mother was chronically depressed most of her life. Whenever I misplace something or forget something I should have remembered, I get scared that I might be mentally ill after all. Whenever I get a headache I wonder if I'm developing a brain tumour."[3]

MERCURY

Mercuriphobia (NP) — From Latin *Mercurius* meaning the Roman god of tradesmen and thieves. Mercury is a poison when swallowed, inhaled or absorbed through the skin.

MESMERISM

See Hypnosis — Hypnophobia.

METAL

Metallophobia (TP) — From Greek *metallo* meaning "metal". German composer Robert Schumann was terrified of metal objects, including keys. He was also phobic of heights and drugs.[4]

METEORS

Meteorophobia (NP) — From Greek *meteoro* meaning "lofty or heavenly body".

MICE

Musophobia (AP) — From Latin *mus* meaning "mouse". Less preferred terms are Muriphobia, Murophobia and Suriphobia. English–US actor Boris Karloff, famous for portraying horror movie characters such as Frankenstein's monster and the Mummy, was afraid of mice. Even more ironic is the fact that Walt Disney, creator of the most commercially successful cartoon character of all time, Mickey Mouse, was actually fearful of mice.[5]

MICROBES

    See **Bacilli** — Bacillophobia.

MICROORGANISM

    See **Bacilli** — Bacillophobia.

MIDGETS

    See **Dwarfs** — Nanosophobia.

MIGRAINES

    See **Headaches** — Hemicraniaphobia.

MIGRATION

    See **Moving (Relocation)** — Tropophobia.

MILK

    Lactophobia (NP) — From Latin *lac* meaning "milk".

MIME ARTISTS

    See **Clowns** — Coulrophobia.

MIND (CONSCIOUS)

    See **Mind (The Mind)** — Psychophobia.

MIND (PRECONSCIOUS)

    See **Mind (The Mind)** — Psychophobia.

MIND (THE MIND)

    Psychophobia (BP) — From Greek *psyche* meaning "mind". This includes fear of the mind (conscious), mind (preconscious), mind (unconscious), mind control and mind reading.

    Case: "I have a phobia I think about quite often, and I am really quite nervous about it. I have a fear that everybody can read my mind all the time, so I never want to think anything personal. The only time when my mind is unreadable is when there is a tinfoil hat on my head. Also, I am afraid that everybody in the world is an actor, and everybody is just making a huge joke out of me. I know that none of these are true, but I can't help but be afraid of them. I believe this may have to do with obsessive-compulsive disorder (OCD), where a thought enters your mind and you can't get rid of it."[6]

MIND (UNCONSCIOUS)

See Mind (The Mind) — Psychophobia.

MIND CONTROL

See Mind (The Mind) — Psychophobia.

MIND READING

See Mind (The Mind) — Psychophobia.

MINIMALISM

Minimalphobia (CP) — From Latin *minimum* meaning "smaller to smallest". This includes fear of downsizing.

MINISTERS

See Religion — Theophobia.

MIRRORS

Eisoptrophobia (TP) — From Greek *eisoptro* meaning "mirror". This includes fear of looking in a mirror, reflection (another's) and reflection (one's own). Less preferred terms are Catoptrophobia, Dysmorphobia and Spectrophobia. US actress Pamela Anderson allegedly suffers from this phobia.

Case: A 48-year-old woman says, "I have always been afraid of my reflection in the mirror. Who is this person? I had an identical twin born after me but she was sickly and weak and died after only a few days. I have always been terrified that the person in the mirror is my dead sister. When I was a girl I sometimes thought that she wanted to exchange bodies with me. If I stood too close to the mirror, she'd pull me in. I avoided mirrors. I still do but not as much as before."[7]

MIRTH

See **Happiness (Being Happy)** — Cherophobia.

MISCARRIAGE

See **Abortion** — Abortivuphobia.

MISSILES

See **Bullets** — Ballistophobia.

MISTAKES

See **Errors** — Hamartophobia.

MISTS

See **Fog** — Homichlophobia.

MITES

Acarophobia (AP) — From Greek *akaris* meaning "a mite".
Less preferred terms are Entomophobia, Insectophobia and
Isopterophobia.

MITRAL VALVE PROLAPSE

MVP-phobia (BP) — From modern terms, "MVP" is an acronym
for the medical condition of mitral valve prolapse.

MOBILITY

See **Walking** — Basiophobia.

MOBS

See **Crowds** — Ochlophobia.

MODELS

See **Statues** — Statuophobia.

MOISTURE

See **Water** — Hydrophobia.

MOLES

Soricomorphapaphobia (AP) — From Greek *soricomorpho* meaning "one that digs and tunnels". This includes fear of gophers.

MONEY

Chrematophobia (TP) — From Greek *chrema* meaning "money". This includes fear of banks. Less preferred terms are Aurophobia and Chrometophobia.

MONITORED (BEING MONITORED)

Monitorphobia (SP) — From Latin *monitor* meaning "one who reminds, admonishes or checks". This includes fear of bugged (being bugged), looked at (being looked at), scrutinised (being scrutinised), seen (being seen), spied upon (being spied upon), stared at (being stared at), surveyed (being surveyed) and surveillance (being under surveillance). Less preferred terms are Ophthalmophobia, Scopophobia and Scoptophobia.

Case: "I know that this is silly, but I have an incredible fear of being stared at. When I leave for work in the morning I feel my neighbours are looking at me. I hate security cameras. I can't stand checking in at an airport and having to go through screening. I often am shaking afterwards. I feel like I've been raped. I grew up in a family that taught, 'Little girls should always be good as God is always watching you'. I believed this. I'm an atheist now but I feel that someone *is* watching me. I know it's silly. I guess I became paranoid when I was a little girl."

* * *

DO HUMANS HAVE AN INNATE FEAR OF BEING STARED AT?
Evidence suggests that humans may be innately fearful of being stared at. This may have evolved as a survival skill. Anthropologists reason that it may be very wise to be "on alert" when being eyed by a hostile

person or possible predator. Studies, beginning in 1965, have shown that social action is stimulated when a person merely sees a pair of eyes looking at them. The human infant is very attentive to the eyes of another person; it is the feature of the face they recognise first. Very early in life the social action produced by being stared at is a fear response.[8]

⋆ ⋆ ⋆

MONKEYS
See Apes — Primatephobia.

MONOTONY
See Boredom — Forarephobia.

MONSTERS
Teratrophobia (CP) — From Greek *teratos* meaning "monster or malformation". Less preferred terms are Dysmorphophobia and Teratophobia.

MOON (THE MOON)
Lunaphobia (NP) — From Latin *luna* meaning "moon". This includes fear of moonlight. A less preferred term is Selenophobia.

MOONLIGHT
See Moon (The Moon) — Lunaphobia.

MOOSE
See Deer — Alkephobia.

MOTHERS
Materaphobia (SP) — From Latin *mater* meaning "mother".

MOTHERS-IN-LAW
Pentheraphobia (SP) — From Greek *penthera* meaning "mother-in-law". Less preferred terms are Novercaphobia and Soceraphobia.

MOTHS

> **Mottephobia** (AP) — From Latin *mot* meaning "movement". Nicole Kidman and Nicola McLean allegedly suffer from this phobia.[9]

MOTION

> **See Movement** — Kinesophobia.

MOTORCYCLES

> **See Cars** — Autokinetophobia.

MOTORCYCLES (BEING A PASSENGER ON A MOTORCYCLE)

> **See Cars (Being a Passenger in a Car)** — Motorphobia.

MOTORCYCLES (DRIVING A MOTORCYCLE)

> **See Cars (Driving a Car)** — Mobilophobia.

MOTORS

> **See Machines** — Mechanophobia.

MOUNTAIN CLIMBING

> **See High Places** — Acrophobia.

MOUNTAIN LIONS

> **See Panthers** — Panther-phobia.

MOUNTAINS

> **See High Places** — Acrophobia.

MOUTH

> **Oralisiphobia** (BP) — From Latin *oralis* meaning "mouth".

MOVEMENT

> **Kinesophobia** (NP) — From Greek *kinesis* meaning "movement". This includes fear of motion. Less preferred terms are Kinessophobia, Kinetophobia, Metathesiophobia and Tropophobia.

MOVING (RELOCATION)

Tropophobia (BP) — From Greek *tropos* meaning "a turn". This includes fear of migration. Less preferred terms are Kinesophobia, Kinessophobia, Kinetophobia and Metathesiophobia.

MOVING VEHICLE (BEING IN A MOVING VEHICLE)

Ochophobia (TP) — From Greek *ocho* meaning "holding".

MUCUS

Blennophobia (NP) — From Greek *blennos* meaning "mucus". This includes fear of slime. A less preferred term is Myxophobia.

MUGGERS

See Bad People — Scelerophobia.

MULTIPLE SEXUAL PARTNERS

Polyiterophobia (SP) — From Greek *poly* meaning "many" and *iteros* meaning "repeat again". *Iteros* is perhaps borrowed from Latin *iterare* meaning "to repeat". The opposite of this phobia is Polyiterophilia, the sexual attraction to multiple sexual partners.

MURDER (ANOTHER'S)

Homocidephobia (SP) — From Latin *homo* meaning "human" and *cidium* meaning "a killing".

MURDER (ONE'S OWN)

Autoassassinophobia (SP) — From Greek *auto* meaning "self" and *assassin* meaning "murderous". *Assass* is perhaps borrowed from Arabic *assassin* meaning "hashish user". The opposite of this phobia is Autoassassinophilia, the sexual attraction to one's own murder.

MURDERERS

See Bad People — Scelerophobia.

MURMURING

See Voice (Another's) — Voxiphobia.

MUSCULAR UNCOORDINATION

See Ataxia — Ataxiaphobia.

MUSEUMS

Museumophobia (CP) — From Latin *museum* meaning "library or study".

Case: "I live in Toronto and there is a museum called the Royal Ontario Museum. I used to have no problem going there until a camp counsellor told a story about the time that [the mummy of] King Tutankhamun of Egypt was supposedly there. I now know it was all a hoax, but I am thoroughly frightened of the entire third floor (where the Egypt exhibit is) and the basement (where the camp counsellor told me the museum kept dead bodies)."[10]

MUSHROOMS

Mycophobia (NP) — From Greek *mycus* meaning "fungus".

MUSIC

Melophobia (CP) — From Greek *melos* meaning "song". A less preferred term is Musicophobia. The opposite of this phobia is Melophilia, the sexual attraction to music.

MYTHS

Mythophobia (CP) — From Greek *mythos* meaning "myth or legend". This includes fear of everything one is told, false statements, lies, lying and stories.

Chapter 13
Phobias Starting with N & O

"We are largely the playthings of our fears. In one, fear of the dark; to another, of physical pain; to a third, of public ridicule; to a fourth, of poverty; to a fifth, of loneliness — for all of us our particular creature awaits us in ambush."

Horace Walpole (1717–1797), *Letters*

NAILS (FINGERS OR TOES)

Onychophobia (BP) — From Greek *onycho* meaning "nails". This includes fear of fingernails and toenails.

NAILS (INDUSTRIAL)

See Pointed Objects — Aichmophobia.

NAKED BODY

See Nudity — Gymnophobia.

NAMED (BEING NAMED)

Onomatophobia (SP) — From Greek *onoma* meaning "name".

NAMES

Nomenatophobia (SP) — From Latin *nomen* meaning "name". This includes fear of hearing a particular name and naming. Less preferred terms are Nomatophobia and Onomatophobia. A legend in the history of science has it that 1905 Nobel Prize for Physics winner Philipp Lenard (1862–1947) suffered such an intense phobia of the name "Isaac Newton" that when he lectured he had to turn his back and have the name written on the blackboard for him. Lenard had a problem with another luminary in physics, Albert Einstein. During the Nazi era, Hungarian–German Lenard denounced Einstein's theory of relativity as "a Jewish fraud".[1]

NAMING

See Names — Nomenatophobia.

NARCOLEPSY

Narcolepsiphobia (BP) — From Greek *narke* meaning "numbness or stupor" and *lepsis* meaning "an attack or seizure". Narcolepsy is a medical condition characterised by excessive daytime sleepiness.

NARROW PLACES AND THINGS

Stenophobia (NP) — From Greek *steno* meaning "narrow". Less preferred terms are Anginaphobia and Anginophobia.

NARROWNESS

Anginophobia (NP) — From Greek *angino* meaning "narrow passage". Less preferred terms are Anginaphobia and Stenophobia.

NAUSEA

Nauseaphobia (BP) — From Greek *nausea* meaning "seasickness". Nausea is a medical condition characterised by stomach unease and discomfort, with the urge to vomit.

NAVEL

Umbilicuphobia (BP) — From Latin *umbilicus* meaning "the navel".

NAZISM

Nazismphobia (CP) — From German *nazi*, which is an abbreviation of *nationalsozialist* based on Old German *sozi* meaning "socialist". It can refer to fear of Nazi doctrine, gatherings, people, rituals or anything else Nazi.

NEEDLES

Belonophobia (TP) — From Greek *belono* meaning "needle".

NEGLECT OF DUTY

Paralipophobia (SP) — From Greek *paraleipein* meaning "to leave aside". This includes fear of neglect of obligations, neglect of responsibility and neglect of work. Less preferred terms are Hypegiaphobia, Hypengyophobia, Paraleipophobia and Paraliphobia.[2]

NEGLECT OF OBLIGATIONS

See Neglect of Duty — Paralipophobia.

NEGLECT OF RESPONSIBILITY

See Neglect of Duty — Paralipophobia.

NEGLECT OF WORK

See Neglect of Duty — Paralipophobia.

NETHERLANDS (THE NETHERLANDS)

See Dutch (The Dutch) — Dutchphobia.

NEW (ANYTHING NEW)

Neophobia (NP) — From Greek *neos* meaning "new". This includes fear of change, innovation, newness, novelty and unfamiliar (the unfamiliar). Less preferred terms are Caenotophobia, Cainophobia, Cainotophobia, Cenophobia, Centophobia, Kainolophobia, Kainophobia, Kainotophobia, Metathesiophobia and Tropophobia. Psychologist, philosopher and futurist Dr Robert Anton Wilson (1932–2007) suggested that Neophobia is deeply ingrained in humans, particularly adults. This accounts for why ideas do not advance as rapidly as does technology.[3]

* * *

DO HUMANS HAVE AN INNATE FEAR OF THE NEW?
Human children show a mixture of fear and fascination with novelty.
Classic experiments by C.W. Vallentine in the 1930s demonstrated
that "fear-fascination" was firmly present in humans by the age of
12 months. On the one hand, something new is unknown and thus may
harm us. On the other, we could learn from it, be helped by it, and it
could even give us pleasure.[4]

* * *

NEWNESS

See New (Anything New) — Neophobia.

NEWTS

Pleurodeliphobia (AP) — From Latin *pleurodelinae* meaning
"newts".

NIGHT

Nyctophobia (NP) — From Greek *nyktos* meaning "night". This
includes fear of dusk and nightfall. Less preferred terms are
Achluophobia, Lygophobia, Myctophobia, Nectophobia and
Noctiphobia.

NIGHTFALL

See Night — Nyctophobia.

NIGHTMARES

See Dreams — Oneirophobia.

NOISES

Ligyrophobia (NP) — From Greek *ligyr* meaning "sharp or
distinct". This includes fear of loud noises and soft noises. Less
preferred terms are Acousticophobia and Phonophobia. Johann
Wolfgang von Goethe and Federico Fellini were terrified of loud
noises, as is Sheryl Crow allegedly.[5]

NON-CLOTHING FABRICS

See Fabrics (Non-clothing) — Hyphephobia.

NON-HUMAN PRIMATES

See Apes — Primatephobia.

NORMALCY

See Conformity — Normophobia.

NORTH AMERICA (THINGS NORTH AMERICAN)

North Amerophobia (CP) — From Old English *nord* meaning "from above" and Latin *Americanus* meaning "the land of America".

NORTHERN LIGHTS

See Auroras — Auroraphobia.

NOSEBLEEDS

Epistaxiophobia (BP) — From Greek *epistaxis* meaning "a dripping (especially related to blood)". Epistaxis is the medical term for a nosebleed.

NOSES

Nasophobia (BP) — From Latin *nasus* meaning "nose". A less preferred term is Rhinophobia. The opposite of this phobia is Nasophilia, the sexual attraction to the nose of a sexual partner.

NOSTALGIA

See Old Things — Retrophobia.

NOTHING

Nilhilophobia (NP) — From Latin *nil* meaning "nothing".

NOVELTY

See New (Anything New) — Neophobia.

NUCLEAR DISASTERS

See Atomic Energy and Science — Atomosophobia.

NUCLEAR ENERGY AND SCIENCE

See Atomic Energy and Science — Atomosophobia.

NUCLEAR EXPLOSIONS

See Atomic Energy and Science — Atomosophobia.

NUCLEAR POWER PLANTS

See Atomic Energy and Science — Atomosophobia.

NUCLEAR WAR

See Atomic Energy and Science — Atomosophobia.

NUCLEAR WEAPONS

See Atomic Energy and Science — Atomosophobia.

NUDITY

Gymnophobia (SP) — From Greek *gymnos* meaning "naked". This includes fear of the naked body. A less preferred term is Nudophobia.

NUISANCES

Nocerephobia (NP) — From Latin *nocere* meaning "to hurt".

NUMBERS

Numerophobia (CP) — From Latin *numer* meaning "number". This includes fear of even numbers, mathematics and odd numbers. A less preferred term is Arithmophobia.

Case: "I have found that I and many other people have a fear of odd numbers. I always turn my TV volume to an even number. I refuse to sign a list if I will be an odd number. Some people do things twice to avoid doing them an odd number of times (turning the light switch off twice, washing hands twice). If I have an odd amount of money I will give away a dollar or something. I am afraid something bad will happen to me on odd-numbered days. Lots of things like that."[6]

NURSING MOTHERS

See Breast-feeding — Lactaphobia.

OATS

Atanphobia (NP) — From Latin *atan* meaning "oats".

OBESITY

Obesophobia (BP) — From Latin *obesitas* meaning "fatness or corpulence". This includes fear of fat (being fat), overweight (being overweight) and weight gain. Less preferred terms are Barophobia, Obesophobia and Pocrescophobia.

OBSESSIONS

Obsessiophobia (CP) — From Latin *obsessus* meaning "besiege or occupy".

OBSESSIVE-COMPULSIVE DISORDER

OCD-phobia (BP) — From modern terms, "OCD" is an acronym for the medical condition of obsessive-compulsive disorder.

OBLIGATIONS

Obligatiophobia (SP) — From Latin *obligation* meaning "pledging".

OBLIVION

Obliviophobia (CP) — From Latin *oblivionem* meaning "utterly forgotten".

OCEANS

See Seas — Thalassophobia.

ODD NUMBERS

See Numbers — Numerophobia.

ODOUR (ANOTHER'S)

See Body Odour (Another's) — Dysomophobia.

ODOUR (ONE'S OWN)

See Body Odour (One's Own) — Autodysomophobia.

ODOUR EMBARRASSMENT (ANOTHER'S)

See Body Odour Embarrassment (Another's) —
Bromidrosiphobia.

ODOUR EMBARRASSMENT (ONE'S OWN)

See Body Odour Embarrassment (One's Own) —
Osphresiophobia.

ODOURS (CERTAIN)

Olfactophobia (NP) — From Latin *olfacto* meaning "smell". This
includes fear of smells. Less preferred terms are Bromidrophobia,
Bromidrosiphobia, Chromatophobia, Chromophobia, Osmophobia
and Osphresiophobia. Dr Benjamin Rush wrote of Olfactophobia:
"The Odor phobia is a very frequent disease with all classes of people.
There are few men or women to whom some smells of some kind
are not disagreeable. Old cheese has often produced paleness and
tremor in a full-fed guest. There are odors from certain flowers that
produce the same effects: hence it is not altogether a figure to say,
that there are persons who 'die of a rose in aromatic pain'."[7]

OLD (BEING OLD)

See Elderly (Being Elderly) — Gerascophobia.

OLD PEOPLE

See Elderly People — Gerontophobia.

OLD THINGS

Retrophobia (NP) — From Latin *retro* meaning "back, backward or
behind". This includes fear of nostalgia.

ONE THING

Monophobia (NP) — From Greek *mono* meaning "single or alone".

ONESELF (BEING BY ONESELF)

See Alone (Being Alone) — Eremophobia.

ONIONS

See Garlic — Alliumphobia.

OPEN HIGH PLACES

Aeroacrophobia (NP) — From Greek *aer* meaning "air" and *acro* meaning "highest".

OPEN SPACES

See Public Places — Agoraphobia.

OPERATING

See Work — Ergasiophobia.

OPINIONS

Doxophobia — From Greek *doxo* meaning "opinion or belief". This includes fear of expressing an opinion. A less preferred term is Allodoxaphobia.

OPPOSING OPINIONS

Allodoxaphobia (SP) — From Greek *allos* meaning "other" and *doxo* meaning "opinion or belief". This includes fear of expressing opposing opinions. A less preferred term is Doxophobia.

OPPOSITE SEX (THE OPPOSITE SEX)

See Heterosexuality — Heterophobia.

ORANGE (COLOUR OR WORD)

Auranjaphobia (NP) — From Greek *auranj* meaning "orange". A less preferred term is Chrysophobia.

ORCHIDS

Orchidophobia (NP) — From Greek *orkhis* meaning "orchid or testicle".

ORDER

Ordinemophobia (SP) — From Latin *ordinem* meaning "row, rank, series, arrangement". This includes fear of orderliness.

ORDERLINESS

See Order — Ordinemophobia.

ORGASMS

See Coitus — Coitophobia.

OSTRICHES

Strouthiophobia (AP) — From Greek *strouthion* meaning "ostrich".

Case: A 34-year-old woman who suffers from this phobia says, "For the longest time now I have had a fear of ostriches. I don't know how it started but I am terrified of them now. Since they aren't common this fear isn't such a big deal but whenever I see them on TV or in a magazine I start screaming or crying. On two different occasions I have burst into tears in museums because I am terrified of the stuffed ostriches in the bird section. Does anyone else find them scary?"[8]

OTTERS

See Furry Aquatic Animals — Lutraphobia.

OUT OF CONTROL (BEING OUT OF CONTROL)

See Control — Contrarotaphobia.

OUTER SPACE

See Space Travel — Spacephobia.

OUTRAGEOUS PEOPLE

See Criminals — Hybristophobia.

OVEREATING

Gluttonophobia (BP) — From Latin *gluttonem* meaning "overeater".

OVERWEIGHT (BEING OVERWEIGHT)

See Obesity — Obesophobia.

OVERWORKING

See Work — Ergasiophobia.

OWLS

Ululaphobia (AP) — From Latin *ulula* meaning "owl". US rapper Eminem allegedly suffers from this phobia.[9]

Chapter 14
Phobias Starting with P

"Fear is kind of a bell ... it is the soul's signal for rallying."
Henry Ward Beecher (1813–1887), *Summer of the Soul*

PAIN (ANOTHER'S)

Torturophobia (SP) — From Latin *tortura* meaning "twisting or torment". Less preferred terms are Agliophobia, Algiophobia, Algophobia, Ergasiophobia, Ergophobia, Odynephobia, Odynophobia and Ponophobia. The opposite of this phobia is Torturophilia, the sexual attraction to inflicting pain on a sexual partner.

PAIN (ONE'S OWN)

Algophobia (BP) — From Greek *algo* meaning "pain". This includes fear of torture (being tortured). Less preferred terms are Agliophobia, Algiophobia, Ergasiophobia, Ergophobia, Odynephobia, Odynophobia, Ponophobia and Torturophobia. Some argue that the most common phobia of all is the fear of pain. Others are not so sure. The opposite of this phobia is Algophilia, the sexual attraction to receiving pain from a sexual partner.

Case: A 25-year-old man says, "I am terrified of pain. Anything but pain. I try to hide it from my mates. If they only knew ..."

PAINTINGS

See Pictures — Pictophobia.

PALINDROMES

Aibohphobia (CP) — From a modern term, "Aibohphobia" is "phobia" spelled backwards and arranged as a palindrome.

PANIC

Panicophobia (BP) — From Greek *panikon* meaning "pertaining to the god Pan".

PANTHERS

Panther-phobia (AP) — From Greek *panther* meaning "tiger". This includes fear of catamounts, cougars, mountain lions and pumas.

PAPER

Papyrophobia (TP) — From Greek *papyros* meaning "paper-reed".

Case: "I am not sure what this would come under, but I have a fear of paper, but not a whole piece of paper. I can handle a piece of paper, but once someone tears it up and crumples it up into little balls, I can't even look at it. I can also take wrappers off things, like candy or straws, but afterwards it can't be in my view or I will vomit. I also can't watch TV if there are paper-towel commercials when they put the towels in the water to wash off the dish. I also have to use a lot of Kleenex, toilet paper or napkins because I can't handle it used or wet. Do you have any idea? Or where I can ask to find out what this phobia is? Or am I just insane?"[1]

PARADOXES

Paradoxophobia (CP) — From Greek *para* meaning "besides, near, from, against or contrary to" and *doxo* meaning "opinion or belief".

PARANOIA

Paranoiaphobia (CP) — From Greek *para* meaning "besides, near, from, against or contrary to" and *noos* meaning "mind". "Paranoia" is itself the Greek word for "mental derangement or madness".

PARASITES

Parasitiophobia (NP) — From Greek *parasitos* meaning "parasite". Less preferred terms are Mysophobia and Parasitophobia. A parasite may be flora or fauna.

PARENTING

Personaliparentephobia (SP) — From Latin *personalis* meaning "pertaining to a person" and *parentum* meaning "ancestor, father or mother".

PARENTS

Parentephobia (SP) — From Latin *parentum* meaning "ancestor, father or mother".

PARENTS-IN-LAW

Soceraphobia (SP) — From Latin *soceri* meaning "parent-in-law". Less preferred terms are Novercaphobia and Pentheraphobia.

PARTIES

See Social Situations — Sociophobia.

PASSING HIGH BUILDINGS

See High Buildings — Batophobia.

PASSING HIGH OBJECTS

See High Buildings — Batophobia.

PASSWORDS

Friend-or-phobia (CP) — From modern terms, "Friend-or-phobia" is a pun referring to "friend-or-foe". This includes fear of bank passwords and computer passwords.[2]

PEANUT BUTTER

Arachibutyrophobia (TP) — From Greek *arakis* meaning "a leguminous plant" and *boutyron* meaning "butter". This includes fear of peanut butter sticking to the roof of the mouth.

PEANUT BUTTER STICKING TO THE ROOF OF THE MOUTH
See Peanut Butter — Arachibutyrophobia.

PELLAGRA
Pellagraphobia (BP) — From Greek *pell* meaning "skin" and *agra* meaning "seizure". Pellagra is a medical condition characterised by skin eruptions, digestive and nervous problems, and mental disturbances including seizures.

PENISES (ERECT)
Medorthophobia (BP) — From Greek *medortho* meaning "erect penis". This includes fear of erections. A less preferred term is Ithyphallophobia.

PENISES (NON-ERECT)
Phallophobia (BP) — From Greek *phallos* meaning "a penis". This includes fear of genitals (male), male genitals and phallic symbols. A less preferred term is Kolpophobia. The opposite of this phobia is Phallophilia, the sexual attraction to the penis size of a sexual partner.

PEOPLE
See Human Beings — Anthropophobia.

PERFECTION
Perfectuphobia (CP) — From Latin *perfectus* meaning "completed".

PERFORMING
See Stage (The Stage) — Topophobia.

PESTILENCE
See Plague — Plagaphobia.

PHALLIC SYMBOLS
See Penises (Non-erect) — Phallophobia.

PHANTOM LIMB SYNDROME

PLS-phobia (BP) — From modern terms, "PLS" is an acronym for the medical condition of phantom limb syndrome.

PHANTOMS

See Spectres — Spectrophobia.

PHILOSOPHY

Philosophobia (CP) — From Greek *phileein* meaning "to love" and *sophia* meaning "wisdom".

PHOBIA (THE WORD)

See Fears — Phobophobia.

PHOBIAS

See Fears — Phobophobia.

PHOTOGRAPHS (ANOTHER'S)

See Pictures — Pictophobia.

PHOTOGRAPHS (ONE'S OWN)

See Pictures — Pictophobia.

PHOTOGRAPHS (THINGS OR OBJECTS)

See Pictures — Pictophobia.

PHYSICAL LOVE

See Eroticism — Erotophobia.

PICNICS

Vuteuthindionophobia (SP) — From Greek *vuteuthindio* meaning "collection of people for eating and pleasure".

PICTURES

Pictophobia (TP) — From Latin *picture* meaning "picture or painting". This includes fear of paintings, photographs (another's), photographs (one's own) and photographs (things or objects).

The opposite of this phobia is Pictophilia, the sexual attraction to paintings, photographs or pictures. Famed English writer Virginia Woolf was terrified of being photographed.[3]

PIGS

Porcuphobia (AP) — From Latin *porcus* meaning "pig or swine". English actor Orlando Bloom is allegedly frightened of pigs. According to one report, when a pig "got loose on the set of *Kingdom of Heaven*, Bloom turned and ran like crazy".[4]

PILLOWS

See Beds — Clinophobia.

PINS

Enetophobia (TP) — From Greek *enetos* meaning "pin". Less preferred terms are Aichmophobia, Belonelphobia and Belonophobia.

PINWHEELS

See Pointed Objects — Aichmophobia.

PIPE SMOKING

See Smoking — Smykheinophobia.

PIPES (HOLLOW)

See Tunnels — Tubuphobia.

PIPES (SOLID)

Piparephobia (TP) — From Latin *pipare* meaning "to peep".

PIPES (TOBACCO)

See Smoking — Smykheinophobia.

PLACES (SPECIFIC PLACES)

Locusaphobia (CP) — From Latin *locus* meaning "place". A less preferred term is Topophobia.

PLAGUE

Plagaphobia (NP) — From Latin *plaga* meaning "pestilence". This includes fear of pestilence.

PLAINS

See Public Places — Agoraphobia.

PLANS (DEFINITE PLANS)

Plannumaphobia (CP) — From Latin *plannum* meaning "level or flat surface". A less preferred term is Teleophobia.

PLANTS

Botanophobia (NP) — From Greek *botanikos* meaning "of herbs". This includes fear of bushes, house plants and shrubs. The pioneering psychoanalyst Sigmund Freud was afraid of house plants, such as ferns. Christina Ricci reportedly will not decorate her house with them and "swears she's afraid of house plants. 'They are dirty,' she said. 'If I have to touch one, after already being repulsed by the fact that there is a plant indoors, then it just freaks me out.'"[5]

PLEASURE

Hedonophobia (BP) — From Greek *hedone* meaning "pleasure". Woody Allen allegedly suffers from this phobia.[6]

POETRY

Metrophobia (CP) — From Greek *metron* meaning "a measure".

POINTED OBJECTS

Aichmophobia (TP) — From Greek *aichme* meaning "the point of a spear". This includes fear of forks, knives, nails (industrial), pinwheels, points, sharp objects and swords. Less preferred terms are Aichurophobia, Apokophobia, Belonephobia, Belonophobia and Enetophobia. James I of England was apparently terrified of an unsheathed sword. French surgeon Antoine Le Camus noted that this fear in James I was the reason for the contemporary comment that "Elizabeth was King, James I was Queen".

Case: A 60-year-old man has been afraid of pointed objects throughout his life. He prefers the forks on the dinner table to be turned upside down. He is very uncomfortable walking near trees during winter; the leaves have fallen and the tiny points of branches are exposed. He believes that pointed objects will become animated and push into his eyes.[7]

POINTS
See Pointed Objects — Aichmophobia.

POISON
Toxicophobia (NP) — From Greek *toxikon* meaning "poison". This includes fear of poison (being poisoned). Less preferred terms are Iophobia, Toxiphobia and Toxophobia. Woody Allen is terrified of being poisoned. He is unable to eat food unless it has been carefully vetted by an elaborate ritual.[8]

POISONED (BEING POISONED)
See Poison — Toxicophobia.

POLAND (THINGS POLISH)
Poloniaphobia (CP) — From Latin *Polonia* meaning "the land of Poland". A less preferred term is Polandophobia.

POLECATS
See Weasels — Galeophobia.

POLES
Polonophobia (TP) — From Latin *palus* meaning "stake".

POLICE
Policiphobia (SP) — From Latin *politia* meaning "civil administration". Alfred Hitchcock was said to have been so

terrified of police as a boy that he later avoided driving a car so that he would never receive a traffic ticket and thus never have to face a police officer.

Case: A 61-year-old man is terrified of policemen, security guards and anyone else wearing a blue suit and looking like a police officer. "As an adolescent in Oakland, California, I saw a white policeman blow a black man's head off in cold blood. The black man just stood there with his arms by his side. The policeman shot him right between the eyes from about three yards away. I ducked for cover and the policeman did not see me. If he had, he might have killed me too to eliminate a witness. The next day the newspaper claimed the policeman shot in self-defence. Since then I am very nervous whenever I see policemen or even security guards. When the transit police come onto a bus to check tickets, I get very nervous and get off the bus if I can."[9]

POLIO

Poliosophobia (BP) — From Greek *polio* meaning "grey matter of the brain and spinal cord". This includes fear of infantile paralysis. Poliomyelitis is a medical condition characterised by loss of muscle movement.

POLITICIANS

See Government — Politicophobia.

POLITICS

See Government — Politicophobia.

POLLUTION

Pollutiophobia (TP) — From Latin *pollutio* meaning "defilement".

POLTERGEISTS

See Spectres — Spectrophobia.

PONDS

See **Lakes** — Limnophobia.

POOLS

See **Lakes** — Limnophobia.

POPES

Papaphobia (SP) — From Latin *papa* meaning "father, bishop or patriarch". A less preferred term is Papophobia.

PORNOGRAPHIC PICTURES

Pornophobia (CP) — From Greek *porne* meaning "a prostitute". The opposite of this phobia is Pornophilia, the sexual attraction to pornographic pictures.

PORNOGRAPHIC TEXTS

Narratophobia (CP) — From Latin *narrare* meaning "to narrate". The opposite of this phobia is Narratophilia, the sexual attraction to pornographic texts.

PORPOISES

See **Marine Mammals** — Cetusaphobia.

POSSESSION (BEING POSSESSED)

Possessiophobia (BP) — From Latin *possessinem* meaning "to possess".

POST-CORONARY BYPASS SURGERY

See **Heart Surgery** — Cardiachirurgiaphobia.

POST-TRAUMATIC STRESS DISORDER

PTSD-phobia (BP) — From modern terms, "PTSD" is an acronym for the medical condition of post-traumatic stress disorder.

POSTNATAL DEPRESSION

PND-phobia (BP) — From modern terms, "PND" is an acronym for the medical condition of postnatal depression. This includes fear of postpartum depression.

POSTPARTUM DEPRESSION

See Postnatal Depression — PND-phobia.

POVERTY (ANOTHER'S)

See Beggars — Mendicarephobia.

POVERTY (ONE'S OWN)

Peniaphobia (CP) — From Greek *penes* meaning "a poverty-stricken or destitute person". This includes fear of destitution.

PRAISE

See Approval — Approbarephobia.

PRECIPICES

See Cliffs — Cremnophobia.

PREGNANCY

Maieusiophobia (BP) — From Greek *maieutikos* meaning "to bring forth children". Less preferred terms are Lockiophobia, Parturiphobia and Tocophobia. The opposite of this phobia is Maieusiophilia, the sexual attraction to a pregnant sexual partner.

PREMENSTRUAL SYNDROME

PMS-phobia (BP) — From modern terms, "PMS" is an acronym for the medical condition of premenstrual syndrome.

PRESCRIPTION DRUGS

See Medicines (Prescription) — Opiophobia.

PRIAPISM

Priapisaphobia (BP) — From Greek *Priapos*, son of the gods Dionysus and Aphrodite, and the god of sexual excess. Priapism is a medical condition characterised by a constant erection.

PRIESTS

See Religion — Theophobia.

PROGRESS

Prosophobia (CP) — From Latin *pro* meaning "forward or in front".

PROJECTILES

See Bullets — Ballistophobia.

PROPERTY

See House (Being in a House) — Domatophobia.

PROPRIETY

Orthophobia (CP) — From Greek *ortho* meaning "straight, true, correct or regular".

PROSTITUTES

Cypridophobia (SP) — From Greek *Kypris* meaning "Venus". Venus is the ancient Greek goddess of love. Less preferred terms are Cyprianophobia, Cyprinophobia, Cypriphobia and Pornophobia.

PROTESTANTISM

Protestantophobia (CP) — From Latin *protestantem* meaning "protest". It can refer to fear of Protestant doctrine, gatherings, people, rituals or anything else Protestant.

PSEUDOSCIENTIFIC TERMS

See Scientific Terms — Hellenologophobia.

PSYCHOSIS

See Insanity (One's Own) — Lyssophobia.

PUBERTY

Pubertaphobia (BP) — From Latin *pubertatem* meaning "age of maturity".

PUBIC LICE

Pubicancerphobia (BP) — From Latin *pubis* meaning "pubic hair" and *cancer* meaning "crab". Pubic lice is a sexually transmitted disease.

PUBLIC PLACES

Agoraphobia (SP) — From Greek *agora* meaning "marketplace". This includes fear of crowded public places, crowded spaces, landscapes, open spaces, plains and safe places. A less preferred term is Agyiophobia. The opposite of this phobia is Agoraphilia, the sexual attraction to sexual behaviour in public places. Those who reportedly suffered or are suffering from Agoraphobia include French philosopher and scientist Blaise Pascal, Polish literary figure Boleslaw Prus, Howard Hughes, Canadian–US science-fiction writer H.L. Gold, US actress Marilyn Monroe, Woody Allen, Aretha Franklin, US singer, songwriter and member of The Beach Boys Brian Wilson, US chef Paula Deen, Argentine–English actress Olivia Hussey, US actress Kim Basinger, US actress Daryl Hannah, English singer Peter Robinson (aka Marilyn), US actress Rose McGowan and US actor Macaulay Culkin. As a result of the trauma he suffered during World War II, Gold's Agoraphobia was so severe that for more than two decades he was unable to leave his flat. Hannah allegedly suffers from Agoraphobia but has kept the fact secret for many years, fearing it might adversely affect her career. Hussey has suffered from it all of her life and has attempted to treat it with meditation rather than medication. McGowan, at one period of her life, would only leave her house once a week in the middle of the night. According to one report, Culkin "doesn't like to leave his apartment".

Case: A 24-year-old woman says, "I hate being in public. I feel that everyone is looking at me, judging me and rejecting me. It is a struggle to get dressed in the morning, put on makeup and get out into the world. Sometimes I just want to run away. I also think men are undressing me with their eyes when all I'm doing is walking on the footpath."[10]

PUBLIC SPEAKING

Glossophobia (SP) — From Greek *glosso* meaning "speech or tongue". This includes fear of speaking in public and the tongue itself. Less preferred terms are Halaphobia and Halophobia. Among those who allegedly suffered or are suffering from Glossophobia are third US President Thomas Jefferson, US inventor, scientist and businessman Thomas Edison, English novelist Agatha Christie, Austrian novelist and playwright Elfriede Jelinek, and Kim Basinger. Jefferson wrote the Declaration of Independence and was a man of great literary skills. But he only gave one speech in his life (for his first inauguration as President in 1801) and communicated his legislative proposals solely in writing. As one report notes, Basinger "could hardly speak at the Oscar ceremony" in 1998 when she had to give an acceptance speech. She was supposedly so frightened that she "rehearsed her speech a few days at a run". George Jessell (1898–1981), known for many decades as the "Toastmaster General of the US" for his frequent role as master of ceremonies at public events, observed that "[t]he human brain starts working the moment you are born and never stops until you stand up to speak in public".

Case: "I work in sales. I have for more than 20 years. I can speak to a client one-on-one. No worries. But to speak in front of a large audience at company functions, I'm hopeless. Two eyes centred on me I can handle. Two hundred eyes, I'm gone. I'm afraid of public speaking. I once did a course in how to overcome it and now I'm a little better than before, but it's still there. I think of speaking into a microphone and I start to sweat."[11]

PUMAS

See **Panthers** — Panther-phobia.

PUNISHED (BEING PUNISHED IN PRIVATE)

See **Beaten in Private (Being Beaten in Private)** — Rhabdophobia.

PUNISHED (BEING PUNISHED IN PUBLIC)

See **Beaten in Public (Being Beaten in Public)** — Mastigophobia.

PUNISHMENT (PUNISHMENT IN ALL FORMS)

Poinephobia (SP) — From Latin *poinikos* meaning "punitive". This includes fear of self-punishment. Less preferred terms are Mastigophobia and Rhabdophobia.

PUPPETS

Pupaphobia (TP) — From Greek *pupa* meaning "puppet". This includes fear of dummies, marionettes and dummies (ventriloquist dummies). A less preferred term is Automatonophobia.

PURPLE (COLOUR OR WORD)

Porphyrophobia (NP) — From Greek *porphyra* meaning "purple".

Chapter 15
Phobias Starting with Q & R

"He who fears something gives it power over him."
Moorish proverb

QUADRATIC EQUATIONS

Quadrataphobia (CP) — From Latin *quadraus* meaning "square".

QUARTETS

Quartophobia (SP) — From Latin *quartus* meaning "fourth". A less preferred term is Quadraphobia.

RABBIS

See Religion — Theophobia.

RABBITS

Lagophobia (AP) — From Greek *lagos* meaning "hare". A less preferred term is Leporiphobia.[1]

RABIES

Rabiphobia (BP) — From Latin *rabies* meaning "madness". Less preferred terms are Aquaphobia, Cainophobia, Cynophobia, Hydrophobia, Hydrophobiaphobia, Hydrophobophobia, Kynophobia, Lyssophobia and Nautophobia. Rabies is a medical condition characterised by acute encephalitis (inflammation of the brain) due to a virus that is zoonotic (transmitted by a bite).

Case: "I am a nurse. I saw a film in nursing school of someone
with rabies. Australia is free from rabies. That has not stopped
me from being afraid of being bitten by a rabid animal, desperate
for water but unable to drink, foaming at the mouth, enduring
excruciating pain, going mad and finally dying. A collapse of
the central nervous system is hideous to watch and worse to
experience."

RACCOONS

See Weasels — Galeophobia.

RADIATION (MEDICAL TREATMENTS)

Radiophobia (BP) — From Greek *radio* meaning "radiate". This
includes fear of X-rays.

RADIATION (SUN'S)

See Sun (The Sun) — Heliophobia.

RADICALISM

See Heresy — Hereiophobia.

RADON

Radonophobia (NP) — From Latin *radius* meaning "ray".

RAILWAY LINES

See Trains — Siderodromophobia.

RAILWAY TRACKS

See Trains — Siderodromophobia.

RAILWAYS

See Trains — Siderodromophobia.

RAIN (BEING RAINED ON)

Ombrophobia (NP) — From Greek *ombros* meaning "rain". This
includes fear of rainstorms. A less preferred term is Pluviophobia.

RAINBOWS

Irisophobia (NP) — From Greek *iris* meaning "iris of the eye, iris plant or rainbow".

Case: "All my life I have been afraid of rainbows. When I see one or see one forming, my heart beats faster and I begin to hyperventilate. Sometimes I cry. Sometimes if I see it suddenly I can't help screaming. I have looked up this fear and found no such thing, but I doubt I'm the only one. I propose to call it Iridophobia. Growing up, I was most afraid of the rainbows you see in the mist of the sprinkler on the lawn. I used to shower with my eyes closed for fear that the spray of the shower would create a rainbow. (I was too young to realise this was not possible, though.) I realise now that I'm not just afraid of rainbows, but things in the sky in general, rainbows and the northern lights especially. I get goosebumps looking at the northern lights, because they're like rainbows that move. That freaks the heck out of me! I shouldn't have moved to Alaska!"[2]

RAINSTORMS

See Rain (Being Rained On) — Ombrophobia.

RAMPS

See Stairs — Climacophobia.

RANDOM VIOLENCE

See Violence — Violentiaphobia.

RAPE (BEING RAPED)

See Sexual Assault — Biastophobia.

RAPE (BEING RAPED WHILE A VIRGIN)

Virginitiphobia (SP) — From Latin *virgo* meaning "maiden".

RAPE (PRETENDED RAPE)

Agonophobia (SP) — From Greek *agon* meaning "struggle".
The opposite of this phobia is Agonophilia, the sexual attraction to
situations involving fake rape or pretend struggle.

RATS

Rodentophobia (AP) — From Latin *rodentum* meaning "to gnaw
and eat away". Less preferred terms are Murophobia, Musophobia
and Zemmiphobia. English actor Joe Swash and Nicola McLean
allegedly suffer from this phobia.

Case: A 71-year-old woman says, "I grew up in an old house.
At night you could hear the rats that lived in the attic. My father
would put out traps and poison, but the rats would always come
back. I could hear them scraggling around up there and gnawing at
things when I tried to go to sleep. Sometimes we'd find a dead rat
in the backyard. I used to be very, very afraid of rats. I was scared
they'd eat me or suck out my blood a little at a time."[3]

RAZORS

Xyrophobia (TP) — From Greek *xyro* meaning "razor".

RECTAL DISEASE

Rectophobia (BP) — From Latin *intestinum rectum* meaning
"straight intestine". Less preferred terms are Proctophobia and
Protophobia.

RECTUM

Proctophobia (BP) — From Greek *proktos* meaning "anus".
This includes fear of anus (the anus). Less preferred terms are
Protophobia and Rectophobia.

RED (COLOUR OR WORD)

Ereuthrophobia (NP) — From Greek *erythros* meaning "blushing
or red". This includes fear of red lights. Less preferred terms are

Ereuthophobia, Erthyrophobia, Erythrophobia, Erytophobia and Rhodophobia. Scottish actor Sean Connery allegedly "is afraid to see a red traffic light, his hands grow cold immediately and the fever begins".[4]

RED LIGHTS

See Red (Colour or Word) — Ereuthrophobia.

REFLECTION (ANOTHER'S)

See Mirrors — Eisoptrophobia.

REFLECTION (ONE'S OWN)

See Mirrors — Eisoptrophobia.

REJECTION

Rejectuphobia (SP) — From Latin *rejectus* meaning "to throw back".

Case: "I was hopeless at sports. I was always the last to be chosen for any side in a team sport. More than once neither side wanted me when there were no other boys to choose. I hated that rejection. It hurt very much. Now as a man I can take rejection better, but still it hurts to think about it and I avoid situations where I might be rejected, especially where others can see it. A few years ago I was asked to stand for office in a local government election. I might have won. But I chose not to stand because I feared losing. Public rejection is what I fear most, even more than death, I think."

RELATIVES

Syngenesophobia (SP) — From Greek *syn* meaning "together" and *genesis* meaning "generation".

RELIGION

Theophobia (CP) — From Greek *theos* meaning "god". This includes fear of God or gods, ministers, priests, rabbis, religious leaders and saints. Less preferred terms are Hagiophobia, Hierophobia and Zeusophobia.

RELIGIOUS CEREMONIES

See Ceremonies — Teleophobia.

RELIGIOUS LEADERS

See Religion — Theophobia.

RELIGIOUS OBJECTS

Hierophobia (CP) — From Greek *hieros* meaning "sacred". This includes fear of sacred objects. A less preferred term is Hagiophobia. The opposite of this phobia is Hierophilia, the sexual attraction to religious objects.

Case: "When I was a boy raised as a Catholic, I used to fear that the crucifix would fly down from the altar and run me through like a sword. The image of someone nailed to the cross scared me as a child too. I hated looking at the wounds in the feet especially."

REPROACH

Enissophobia (CP) — From Greek *enisso* meaning "reproach". This includes sin (unpardonable sin). Less preferred terms are Enosiophobia, Hamartophobia, Kritikophobia and Scruptophobia.[5]

REPTILES

Herpetophobia (AP) — From Greek *herpeton* meaning "reptile". This includes fear of alligators, crawling animals, crocodiles and lizards. Less preferred terms are Batrachophobia and Ophidiophobia. English actor and comedian Norman Pace is allegedly frightened of crocodiles. US singer Britney Spears is supposedly terrified of the Komodo dragon.

Case: "There's something about reptiles that is so repulsive! I have nightmares about them. I used to have a recurring nightmare of being chased by a giant lizard, caught and then eaten. It used to scare me. I've never really overcome it. Reptiles are just awful!"[6]

RESPONSIBILITY

Hypengyophobia (SP) — From Greek *hypo* meaning "under" and *engys* meaning "close". This includes fear of accountability and duty. Less preferred terms are Hypaegiaphobia, Hypegiaphobia, Paraliphobia and Paralipophobia.

RETIREMENT

See Elderly (Being Elderly) — Gerascophobia.

RETIREMENT CEREMONIES

See Ceremonies — Teleophobia.

RETURNING

See Home (Returning Home) — Nostophobia.

REVOLVING DOORS

See Doors — Thuraphobia.

RICE

Oryzaphobia (NP) — From Greek *oryza* meaning "rice".

RIDICULE

Catagelophobia (SP) — From Greek *kata* meaning "down" and *gelaein* meaning "laugh". This includes fear of humiliation, laughter (another's) and looking ridiculous. A less preferred term is Katagelophobia.

Case: A 47-year-old man says, "I have had an intense fear of being humiliated in front of a group my whole life. When I was in fifth class in school, I was humiliated by a teacher in front of the whole class. I don't remember what I did to deserve it. I just remember the others laughing at me. I avoid all situations where I might be ridiculed in front of people."[7]

RIGHT (THINGS TO THE RIGHT)
See **Right-handedness** — Dextrophobia.

RIGHT SIDE (THINGS ON THE RIGHT SIDE OF ONE'S OWN BODY)
See **Right-handedness** — Dextrophobia.

RIGHT-HANDEDNESS
Dextrophobia (BP) — From Latin *dexter* meaning "right-handed". This includes fear of the right (things to the right), right side (things on the right side of one's own body) and right-sided objects.

RIGHT-SIDED OBJECTS
See **Right-handedness** — Dextrophobia.

RITUALS
Ritualisiphobia (CP) — From Latin *ritualis* meaning "relating to religious rites".

RIVERS
Potamophobia (NP) — From Greek *potamos* meaning "a river". This includes fear of running water and sheets of water. A less preferred term is Potamphobia.

ROAD RAGE
Road Rage-phobia (SP) — From modern terms, "road rage" is uncontrollable anger when behind the wheel of a motor vehicle.

ROAD TRAVEL
See **Travel** — Hodophobia.

ROBBED (BEING ROBBED)
Chrematistophobia (SP) — From Greek *khrematismos* meaning "money-making". This includes fear of charged for sex (being charged for sex). A less preferred term is Harpaxophobia. The opposite of this phobia is Chrematistophilia, the sexual attraction to being robbed or charged for sex.

ROBBERS

See Bad People — Scelerophobia.

ROBBING

Harpaxophobia (SP) — From Greek *harpax* meaning "to snatch". This includes fear of charging for sex. The opposite of this phobia is Harpaxophilia, the sexual attraction to robbing or charging for sex.

RODS

See Beaten in Private (Being Beaten in Private) — Rhabdophobia.

ROOM FULL OF PEOPLE (A ROOM FULL OF PEOPLE)

See Rooms — Koinoniphobia.

ROOMS

Koinoniphobia (SP) — From Greek *koino* meaning "shared space". This includes fear of crowded rooms and room full of people (a room full of people). A less preferred term is Cenophobia. The great 18th century English author Samuel Johnson suffered from this phobia. He once asked to be excused from jury duty because he came "very near fainting ... in all crowded places".[8]

RUBBER

See Latex — Latexophobia.

RUIN (BEING RUINED)

Atephobia (SP) — From Greek *ate* meaning "rash or destructive deeds". Ate was the Greek goddess of rash and destructive deeds.

RUINS

Ruinaphobia (TP) — From Latin *ruina* meaning "a collapse".

RUNNING WATER

See Rivers — Potamophobia.

RUSSIA (THINGS RUSSIAN)

Russophobia (CP) — From Latin *Russi* meaning "the people of Russia".

RUST

Iophobia (NP) — From Greek *ios* meaning "rust". A less preferred term is Lophobia.

Chapter 16
Phobias Starting with S

"The great source of terror to infancy is solitude. The teleology of this is obvious, as is also that of the infant's expression of dismay — the never failing cry — on waking up and finding himself alone."

William James (1842–1910), *Psychology: The Briefer Course*

SACRED OBJECTS

See Religious Objects — Hierophobia.

SAFE PLACES

See Public Places — Agoraphobia.

SAFETY FROM ONE'S OWN PHOBIAS

See Fear Avoidance — Counterphobia.

SAINTS

See Religion — Theophobia.

SALAMANDERS

Urodelaphobia (AP) — From Latin *urodela* meaning "salamanders".

SALIVA

See Vomiting — Emetophobia.

SALT

Saliphobia (NP) — From Latin *sal* meaning "salt". This includes fear of saltiness.

SALTINESS

See **Salt** — Saliphobia.

SALTY BODY FLUIDS

Salirophobia (BP) — From Latin *sal* meaning "salt". The opposite of this phobia is Salirophilia, the sexual attraction to tasting salty body fluids.

SAME SEX (THE SAME SEX)

See **Homosexuality** — Homophobia.

SAMENESS

See **Boredom** — Forarephobia.

SAND

See **Dust** — Amathophobia.

SATAN

Satanophobia (CP) — From Greek *Satan* meaning "the Devil". This includes fear of devils. Less preferred terms are Demonaphobia, Demoniphobia, Demonophobia and Entheophobia.

SCABIES

Scabiophobia (BP) — From Latin *scabere* meaning "to scratch". Scabies is a medical condition characterised by a parasitic skin infection.

SCHEDULES

See **Time** — Chronophobia.

SCHIZOPHRENIA

Schizophreniphobia (BP) — From Greek *skhizein* meaning "to split" and *phren* meaning "mind". Schizophrenia is a medical condition characterised by abnormalities in the perception or expression of reality.

SCHOOL (GOING TO SCHOOL)

School-phobia (SP) — From Greek *schole* meaning "a school or lecture". Less preferred terms are Didaskaleinophobia and Scholionophobia.[1]

SCIENTIFIC TERMS

Hellenologophobia (CP) — From Greek *hellene* meaning "language". This includes fear of complex scientific terms, cumbersome scientific terms, Greek terms, jargon, pseudoscientific terms and terminology.[2]

SCOTLAND (THINGS SCOTTISH)

Scotophobia (CP) — From Latin *Scotus* meaning "a Scot".

SCOURGED (BEING SCOURGED IN PRIVATE)

See Beaten in Private (Being Beaten in Private) — Rhabdophobia.

SCOURGED (BEING SCOURGED IN PUBLIC)

See Beaten in Public (Being Beaten in Public) — Mastigophobia.

SCRATCHED (BEING SCRATCHED)

Amychophobia (BP) — From Greek *mychia* meaning "a scratch". This includes fear of clawed (being clawed), claws and scratches.

SCRATCHES

See Scratched (Being Scratched) — Amychophobia.

SCRUTINISED (BEING SCRUTINISED)

See Monitored (Being Monitored) — Monitorphobia.

SCRUTINISING

See Watching — Scopophobia.

SEALS

See Furry Aquatic Animals — Lutraphobia.

SEAS

Thalassophobia (NP) — From Greek *thalassa* meaning "the sea".
This includes fear of oceans. Less preferred terms are Nautophobia
and Thalassiophobia. Among those who suffer from this phobia are
Michelle Pfeiffer and Carmen Electra. Although attaining stardom
on surf-rescue TV show *Baywatch*, Electra has confessed to being
afraid of the ocean: "I get terrified anywhere near it and have a
panic attack."

Case 1: "I suppose my weirdest fear is my fear of algae and
coral/coral reefs. It was worse when I was younger but I still
don't like them. The fear is caused by the fact that algae and coral
are alive. I feel like it's watching me. When I was younger I had
nightmares of it watching me and then tangling around me and
trapping/engulfing me."

Case 2: "For as long as I can remember I have been terrified of
the ocean. Not because it's a huge body of water, but because of
octopi and jellyfish and other creatures with suckers and stingers,
not sharks or anything that can actually kill you. One time I was at
the aquarium and had to sit down, so I sat up against the tank that
I thought had fish or something in it. When my friend, who knew
I was terrified of octopi, asked me what I was doing, I said sitting.
She told me to get up slowly and not look back. Being stupid, or
just curious, I looked behind me first. There was a giant octopus
with his mouth right behind my head. In complete panic mode I
leaped up and, unfortunately, so did my lunch. I haven't been to
the shore in years and any time I am near a body of water I begin
to panic heavily."[3]

SEASONAL AFFECTIVE DISORDER

SAD-phobia (BP) — From modern terms, "SAD" is an acronym for
the medical condition of seasonal affective disorder.

SECRETS

Secretuphobia (CP) — From Latin *secretus* meaning "separate, apart or private".

SEDATIVES

See Medicines — Pharmacophobia.

SEEING

See Watching — Scopophobia.

SEEN (BEING SEEN)

See Monitored (Being Monitored) — Monitorphobia.

SELF (THE SELF)

Autophobia (BP) — From Greek *autos* meaning "self". Less preferred terms are Eremophobia and Monophobia.

SELF-PUNISHMENT

See Punishment (Punishment in All Forms) — Poinephobia.

SELF-STRANGULATION

Asphyxiophobia (BP) — From Greek *asphyxia* meaning "stopping of the pulse". The opposite of this phobia is Asphyxiophilia, the sexual attraction to self-strangulation.

SEMEN

See Sperm — Spermatophobia.

SEPARATION

Separarephobia (CP) — From Latin *separare* meaning "divide, distinguish or separate".

SEPULCHRES

See Cemeteries — Coimetrophobia.

SERMONS

Homilophobia (CP) — From Greek *homilia* meaning "a sermon". This includes fear of addresses, lectures and speeches. The opposite of this phobia is Homilophilia, the sexual attraction to sermons or speeches.[4]

SEX

Genophobia (BP) — From Greek *geno* meaning "begetting or producing". This includes fear of libido and sexual fears. A less preferred term is Coitophobia.

SEXUAL ABUSE

Contrectophobia (SP) — From Latin *contrectare* meaning "to handle". Less preferred terms are Agraphobia and Contreltophobia.

SEXUAL ASSAULT

Biastophobia (SP) — From Greek *biastos* meaning "violent". This includes fear of rape (being raped). The opposite of this phobia is Biastophilia, the sexual attraction to sexual assault.

SEXUAL CONTACT INVOLVING THE GENITALS

See Coitus — Coitophobia.

SEXUAL CONTACT INVOLVING THE MOUTH

Coitusoralisiphobia (SP) — From Latin *coitus* meaning "copulation" and *oralis* meaning "mouth".

SEXUAL CONTACT INVOLVING WILD BEASTS

Coitusmoreferaphobia (SP) — From Latin *coitus* meaning "copulation" and *more ferarum* meaning "feral beasts".

SEXUAL FEARS

See Sex — Genophobia.

SEXUAL INTERCOURSE

> **Coitusintercursuphobia (SP)** — From Latin *coitus* meaning "copulation" and *intercursus* meaning "a running between". Less preferred terms are Coitophobia, Cypridophobia and Cypriphobia.

SEXUAL LOVE

> See **Eroticism** — Erotophobia.

SEXUAL PERVERSION

> **Paraphobia (CP)** — From Greek *para* meaning "abnormal and wrong".

SEXUAL QUESTIONS

> See **Eroticism** — Erotophobia.

SEXUALLY TRANSMITTED DISEASES

> **Cypriphobia (BP)** — From Greek *cypri* meaning "lewd". This includes fear of venereal diseases. Less preferred terms are Cyprianophobia, Cypridophobia, Cyprinophobia and Venereophobia.

SHADOWS

> **Sciophobia (NP)** — From Greek *skia* meaning "a shadow". A less preferred term is Sciaphobia.

SHAKING

> See **Trembling** — Tremophobia.

SHALLOTS

> See **Garlic** — Alliumphobia.

SHARP OBJECTS

> See **Pointed Objects** — Aichmophobia.

SHARKS

> **Selachophobia (AP)** — From Greek *selacho* meaning "shark". Less preferred terms are Galeophobia and Gatophobia. Jennifer

Love Hewitt, Christina Ricci, US pop musician and actor Justin Timberlake, and Amanda and Samantha Marchant, known together as "Samanda", are among those who allegedly suffer from this phobia.

Case: A long-time surfer says, "I have been surfing for 30 years. My biggest fear is a shark. I have nightmares about waiting for a wave and seeing a fin in the water going for me. I have had this phobia since I saw *Jaws* years ago."[5]

SHEETS OF WATER

See Rivers — Potamophobia.

SHELLFISH

Ostraconophobia (AP) — From Greek *ostrakon* meaning "shellfish". This includes fear of crabs and lobsters. French philosopher Jean-Paul Sartre suffered from Ostraconophobia; he was terrified of crabs.

Case: "I have a serious fear of lobsters. I can't stand to walk by them in supermarkets or seafood restaurants."[6]

SHIPS

Nautophobia (TP) — From Greek *nautes* meaning "sailor". This includes fear of boats, drowning (drowning while on a boat, ship or vessel) and vessels.

Case: "My fear of large boats in deep water comes from one movie, *The Poseidon Adventure*. Before that, no fear. *Jaws* also lent a bit of additional fear, especially the captain's World War II tale of his buddy's lower half being eaten by a shark. Shudder!"[7]

SHOCK

Hormephobia (BP) — From Greek *hormein* meaning "to stir up".

SHOCK TREATMENT

See Electroconvulsive Therapy — Electroconvulsiphobia.

SHOES

Pedicooperiphobia (TP) — From Latin *pedis* meaning "foot" and *cooperire* meaning "to cover over".

SHOES WITH HIGH HEELS

See Boots — Altocalciphobia.

SHOOTING

See Firearms — Hoplophobia.

SHOPPING

Optarephobia (SP) — From Latin *optare* meaning "desire and choose".

SHORT-LIVED SUCCESS

See Success — Polycratiphobia.

SHOUTING

See Voice (Another's) — Voxiphobia.

SHOWERS (TAKING A SHOWER)

Pluviophobia (BP) — From Latin *pluvio* meaning "rain".

SHRINKING

See Small Objects and Things — Microphobia.

SHRUBS

See Plants — Botanophobia.

SHUT IN (BEING SHUT IN)

See Enclosed Spaces — Claustrophobia.

SIDS

SIDS-phobia (BP) — From modern terms, "SIDS" is an acronym for the medical condition of sudden infant death syndrome.

SILENCE

Sedatephobia (NP) — From Latin *sedentarius* meaning "remaining still".

SILVER

Argentuphobia (NP) — From Latin *argentum* meaning "silver".

SIN

Peccatophobia (CP) — From Latin *peccare* meaning "to sin". Less preferred terms are Enissophobia, Enosiophobia, Hamartophobia, Harmatophobia and Scruptophobia. The opposite of this phobia is Peccatophilia, the sexual attraction to sin, sinning or a sexual partner who sins.

SIN (UNPARDONABLE SIN)

See Reproach — Enissophobia.

SINGAPORE (THINGS SINGAPOREAN)

Maserphobia (CP) — From Greek *mase* meaning "mixed". Singapore is known as a mixed-culture society.

SINGING

See Voice (Another's) — Voxiphobia.

SINGLE (BEING SINGLE)

See Unmarried (Being Unmarried) — Anuptaphobia.

SITTING

Cathisophobia (BP) — From Greek *kata* meaning "down" and *hizein* meaning "to seat". Less preferred terms are Kathisophobia and Thaasophobia.

SITTING STILL

Thaasophobia (BP) — From Greek *thaaso* meaning "sit still".

SIX HUNDRED AND SIXTY-SIX (NUMBER 666)

Hexakosioihexekontahexaphobia (CP) — From Greek *hexakosioihexekontahexa* meaning "the number 666". The number 666 is the number of "the Beast" in the Book of Revelation. It is also the sum of all numbers on a roulette wheel — accounting for the aversion of some to roulette wheels.

SKIN

Dermaphobia (BP) — From Greek *dermatos* meaning "skin".

SKIN DISEASE

Dermatopathophobia (BP) — From Greek *dermatos* meaning "skin" and *pathos* meaning "suffering". This includes skin lesions. Less preferred terms are Dermatophobia and Dermatosiophobia.

SKIN LESIONS

See Skin Disease — Dermatopathophobia.

SKYDIVING

See High Places — Acrophobia.

SLEEP

Somnophobia (BP) — From Latin *somnus* meaning "sleep". This includes fear of sleep talking. Less preferred terms are Hypnophobia and Somniphobia. The opposite of this phobia is Somnophilia, the sexual attraction to sleep or a sexual partner who is asleep.

SLEEP TALKING

See Sleep — Somnophobia.

SLIDING DOWN A DRAINPIPE

See Drains — Suspirarephobia.

SLIME

See Mucus — Blennophobia.

SLIPS OF THE TONGUE

See **Speaking** — Phonophobia.

SLOWNESS

Lentuphobia (NP) — From Latin *lentus* meaning "slow and sluggish".

SMALL ANIMALS

Microbiophobia (AP) — From Greek *mikros* meaning "tiny" and *bios* meaning "life". A less preferred term is Acarophobia.

SMALL OBJECTS AND THINGS

Microphobia (NP) — From Greek *mikros* meaning "tiny". This includes fear of shrinking. Less preferred terms are Mycrophobia and Tapinophobia.

Case: "Have you ever heard of a fear of shrinking? Every now and then I will be in a dream in which I am subjected to a shrink ray or magical shrinking spell and start to get smaller (that is, my surroundings appear to grow). I generally wake up immediately in a cold sweat with heart pounding."[8]

SMALL ROOMS (BEING IN A SMALL ROOM)

See **Enclosed Spaces** — Claustrophobia.

SMALL SPACES (BEING IN A SMALL SPACE)

See **Enclosed Spaces** — Claustrophobia.

SMELLS

See **Odours (Certain)** — Olfactophobia.

SMOKE

See **Fog** — Homichlophobia.

SMOKING

Smykheinophobia (BP) — From Greek *smykhein* meaning "to burn with a smouldering flame". This includes fear of cigar smoking, cigars, cigarette smoking, cigarettes, pipe smoking, pipes and tobacco. Alfred Hitchcock supposedly experienced Smykheinophobia.[9]

SMOTHERING (BEING SMOTHERED)

Pnigerophobia (BP) — From Greek *pnigeros* meaning "smother". A less preferred term is Pnigophobia.

SNAKES

Ophidiophobia (AP) — From Greek *ophis* meaning "snake". Less preferred terms are Herpetophobia, Ophiciophobia, Ophiophobia and Snakephobia. The opposite of this phobia is Ophidiophilia, the sexual attraction to snakes. Those who allegedly have suffered or are suffering from Ophidiophobia include Johnny Cash, Esther Rantzen, Canadian comedian, actor, director and writer David Steinberg, US actor and comedian Chevy Chase, English TV chef Ainsley Harriot, English snooker champion Jimmy White, English model, singer and dancer Samantha Fox, English model Nell McAndrew, Justin Timberlake, Joe Swash, Carly Zucker and Nicola McLean.

Case 1: "I'm deadly afraid of snakes. Even when they are on TV I will just freak out. I have never really thought about trying to conquer it. To be honest, I don't want to. I enjoy being afraid of snakes. I hate how creepy and slimy they look. Just thinking about them makes me cringe."

Case 2: "I hate snakes. They are just slimy and yucky. When I was growing up, my brothers had pythons and other types of snakes, and I just hate them. I also grew up in the country so we had a lot of snakes around the place."[10]

★ ★ ★

DO HUMANS HAVE AN INNATE FEAR OF SNAKES?
Early experiments on whether or not humans have an innate fear
of snakes determined that when a snake is placed before a young
child, they show no fear of snakes until about 24 months of age. By
36 months or so, they show "some caution". Up until this time a snake
may still be touched by the child without apparent fear. But by age
four years, there is "definite fear" seen. Although there are few snake
bites in the UK, two researchers found that one-third of British children
were fearful of snakes at age 14.[11]

* * *

UNLOCKING THE FEAR OF SNAKES (AND SPIDERS TOO)
University of Queensland researchers have discovered evidence that
could help us get to the bottom of the causes of some of our most
common phobias. Hundreds of thousands of people count snakes
and spiders among their greatest fears. Scientists have traditionally
theorised that we possess an evolutionary predisposition to fear such
unfamiliar animals because they may have a greater possibility of
harming us. Nature favours the careful — or so the reasoning goes.
The researchers compared the responses to stimuli of participants
with no particular experience with snakes and spiders to that of snake
and spider experts. It was concluded that "people tend to be exposed
to a lot of negative information regarding snakes and spiders [and]
this makes them more likely to be associated with phobia". They add,
"We showed that although everyone preferentially attends to snakes
or spiders in the environment as they are potentially dangerous, only
inexperienced participants display a negative response." In other
words, the researchers argue that the fear, at least to the degree that
it becomes a phobia, is not innate but learned.[12]

* * *

SNOW

Chionophobia (NP) — From Greek *chion* meaning "snow". This includes fear of ice. Less preferred terms are Cheimaphobia, Cheimatophobia, Cryophobia, Frigophobia, Pagophobia and Psychrophobia.

SOCIAL SITUATIONS

Sociophobia (SP) — From Latin *socius* meaning "a companion". This includes fear of attention, embarrassment, evaluation (being evaluated), examinations (non-academic), parties, society and tests (non-academic). Less preferred terms are Anthropophobia and Social Phobia. Those who allegedly suffered or are suffering from Sociophobia include US novelist and short-story author Nathaniel Hawthorne, Abraham Lincoln, US slavery abolitionist and author Harriet Beecher Stowe, US teacher, nurse, humanitarian and founder of the Red Cross Clara Barton, 18th US President and general Ulysses S. Grant, Irish playwright George Bernard Shaw, 26th US President Theodore Roosevelt, US sharpshooter Annie Oakley, US co-inventor of the aeroplane Orville Wright, US poet Robert Frost, German–US physicist and mathematician Albert Einstein, US First Lady and political figure Eleanor Roosevelt, US industrialist Leroy Grumman, Agatha Christie, US actor Henry Fonda, US comedienne, actress and TV producer Lucille Ball, US singing cowboy and actor Roy Rogers, English actor Sir Alec Guinness, Swedish actress Ingrid Bergman, US jazz singer Ella Fitzgerald, US newspaper publisher Katharine Graham, US comedian and TV personality Johnny Carson, US comedian and actor Don Rickles, US actress Nancy Marchand, US actor Gene Hackman, US astronaut Neil Armstrong, US comedienne, actress and TV personality Joan Rivers, US singer and actor Elvis Presley, Woody Allen, US short-story author and poet Raymond Carver, Swedish–US actress, singer and dancer Ann-Margret, US singer and songwriter Bob Dylan, US actor Harrison Ford, US author, humorist and satirist Garrison Keillor, George Harrison, Robert De Niro, Cher, Elfriede Jelinek, US actress Sally Field, English singer, musician and actor David Bowie, US TV personality David Letterman, Australian actor and comedian Garry McDonald, US radio personality Michael Feldman, US businessman Craig McCaw, Richard Gere, US actress Sigourney Weaver, US Olympic gymnast, actress and TV commentator Cathy Rigby, US jazz singer and pianist Diane Schuur, US model and actress Rene Russo, US actor, director and film producer Kevin Costner, US actor Tom Hanks, Cuban–US singer and songwriter Gloria Estefan, US singer, musician and actor Donny Osmond, US singer Mary Chapin Carpenter, Michelle Pfeiffer, Australian actress Louise Siversen, US activist and environmentalist Erin Brockovich, US children's author Kimberly Willis Holt, Tom Cruise, Canadian–US actor and comedian Jim Carrey, Brad Pitt, US actress Courtney Cox, Australian–New Zealand actress Rebecca Gibney, Nicole Kidman, US actress Julia Roberts, English pop tenor Paul Potts, US soccer player Mia Hamm, Australian swimmer Susie O'Neill, Norah Jones, and US singer and songwriter Carrie Underwood.[13]

★ ★ ★

INCREASED BRAIN ACTIVITY IN SOCIOPHOBIA

Monash University researchers have concluded that up to one in 20 Australians may suffer from some degree of Sociophobia. This makes it the most common anxiety disorder in Australia and the third-most common psychiatric disorder after depression and alcohol dependence. Their research also shows that people suffering generalised Sociophobia experience increased brain activity when confronted with threatening faces or frightening social situations. The researchers found that the area of the brain called the amygdala becomes increasingly hyperactive when patients look at threatening, angry, disgusted or fearful faces. Furthermore, they found that the increased response in the amygdala correlated with the level of the patient's Sociophobia symptoms. The amygdala is in the limbic part of the brain. This basic or primitive part of the brain controls "emotions of threat" and sends messages to the parts of the brain that control breathing and heart rate.[14]

* * *

IS THE BRAIN OF THE SOCIOPHOBE DIFFERENT?
Dutch researchers believe they have detected biochemical differences in the brains of individuals with Sociophobia (also known as generalised social anxiety disorder) thus providing evidence of a long-suspected biological cause for this disorder. Using single photon emission computed tomography to view the brain, the study compared densities of elements of the serotonin and dopamine neurotransmitter systems in the brains of 12 people diagnosed with Sociophobia, but who had not taken medication to treat it, with those of 12 healthy people who were matched by sex and age. Both groups were injected with a radioactive compound that binds with elements of the serotonin and dopamine systems of the brain. Once administered, the radiotracer revealed functional alterations in these brain systems by measuring the radioactive binding in the thalamus, midbrain and pons regions (known to be acted upon by serotonin) and in the striatum region (known to be acted upon by dopamine). The altered uptake activity in these regions indicated a greater level of disordered function.

According to Dr Van der Wee, "Our study provides direct evidence for the involvement of the brain's dopaminergic system in social anxiety disorder in patients who had no prior exposure to medication. It demonstrates that social anxiety has a physical, brain-dependent component." This suggests that the brains of people with Sociophobia may very well be different.[15]

222

* * *

OXYTOCIN MAY SLOW SOCIOPHOBIA

Swedish and British researchers have shown, using functional magnetic resonance imaging (fMRI), that the hormone oxytocin can inhibit feelings of anxiety in specific individuals. Oxytocin is a neuropeptide that is secreted by the body during massage, childbirth and breast-feeding to induce a calming and analgesic effect. Oxytocin has a direct influence on the amygdala. In experiments at the Karolinska Institutet in Stockholm and the Welcome Trust in London, subjects were shown pictures of four different faces, two of which were combined with a tiny, harmless but nevertheless uncomfortable electric shock. As expected, it was found that the faces associated with the shock were considered more unpleasant than the others. However, when half the subjects were then given oxytocin spray and the other half a placebo spray, an interesting change was brought about. When the oxytocin group again saw the two faces that had previously been associated with the shock, they no longer found them disagreeable, while those who had received the placebo still found them so. The researchers concluded that oxytocin has a more targeted effect than simply producing a general feeling of well-being.[16]

* * *

SOCIOPHOBIA SUFFERERS SEE THEMSELVES DIFFERENTLY

Using magnetic resonance imaging (MRI) of the brain, researchers at the US National Institutes of Health have discovered that patients with generalised Sociophobia respond differently from other people to negative comments about themselves. In a series of experiments comparing patients with generalised Sociophobia and those without Sociophobia, those with Sociophobia showed increased blood flow in their medial prefrontal cortex and their amygdala when reading negative statements about themselves. These are areas of the brain linked to concepts of self as well as to fear, emotion and stress response. However, there were no differences between the two groups in their responses to negative comments referring to others, or neutral or positive comments referring to either themselves or others. Previous studies have found differences in the way that brains of affected individuals respond to facial expressions, which suggest that Sociophobia involves increased responsiveness to social stimuli in areas linked to emotion.[17]

★ ★ ★

SOCIALISM

Socialismphobia (CP) — From Latin *socialis* meaning "united or living with others". It can refer to fear of Socialist doctrine, gatherings, people, rituals or anything else Socialist.

SOCIETY

See Social Situations — Sociophobia.

SOFT NOISES

See Noises — Ligyrophobia.

SOFT TALKING

See Voice (Another's) — Voxiphobia.

SOLITUDE

See Alone (Being Alone) — Eremophobia.

SOUNDS

Acousticophobia (NP) — From Greek *akoustikos* meaning "related to sound". This includes fear of echoes. Less preferred terms are Ligyrophobia and Phonophobia. The opposite of this phobia is Acousticophilia, the sexual attraction to sounds.

SOURNESS

Acerophobia (NP) — From Latin *acerbus* meaning "sour, sharp or bitter". A less preferred term is Acerbophobia. This fear leads to the avoidance of acerbic food and drink. Taste, smell, or both of these senses, may be involved.

SOUTH AMERICA (THINGS SOUTH AMERICAN)

South Amerophobia (CP) — From Old English *sud* meaning "from below" and Latin *Americanus* meaning "the land of America".

SOUTHERN LIGHTS

See Auroras — Auroraphobia.

SPACE TRAVEL

Spacephobia (NP) — From Latin *spatium* meaning "room, area, distance or stretch of time". This includes fear of outer space.

SPANKED (BEING SPANKED IN PRIVATE)

See Beaten in Private (Being Beaten in Private) — Rhabdophobia.

SPANKED (BEING SPANKED IN PUBLIC)

See Beaten in Public (Being Beaten in Public) — Mastigophobia.

SPEAKING

Phonophobia (SP) — From Greek *phone* meaning "speech sound". This includes fear of slips of the tongue, speech, speech errors, talking, using the wrong words, verbal slips and voice (one's own). Less preferred terms are Glossophobia, Laliophobia and Lalophobia. US concert promoter David Gest supposedly suffers from this phobia.[18]

SPEAKING IN PUBLIC

See Public Speaking — Glossophobia.

SPEAKING ON THE TELEPHONE

See Telephones — Telephonophobia.

SPECTRES

Spectrophobia (CP) — From Latin *spectrum* meaning "appearance, vision, apparition" or "ghosts and phantoms". This includes fear of angels, ghosts, goblins, phantoms, poltergeists and spirits. Less preferred terms are Bogyphobia, Phasmaphobia, Phasmophobia and Pneumatiphobia. The opposite of this phobia is Spectrophilia, the sexual attraction to angels, ghosts, goblins, phantoms, poltergeists or spirits. Johnny Depp and Christina Ricci supposedly suffer from Spectrophobia.[19]

SPEECH

See Speaking — Phonophobia.

SPEECH ERRORS

See Speaking — Phonophobia.

SPEECHES

See Sermons — Homilophobia.

SPEED

Tachophobia (NP) — From Greek *tachos* meaning "speed".[20]

SPELLING MISTAKES

Ortographobia (CP) — From Greek *orto* meaning "incorrect" and *graphikos* meaning "of or for writing". This includes fear of wrongly chosen letters. A less preferred term is Retterophobia.

SPERM

Spermatophobia (BP) — From Greek *sperma* meaning "seed". This includes fear of semen. Less preferred terms are Spermaphobia and Spermophobia.

SPIDERS

Arachnophobia (AP) — From Greek *arachne* meaning "a spider". A less preferred term is Arachnephobia. The opposite of this phobia is Arachnophilia, the sexual attraction to spiders. Fifty per cent of American women and 10 per cent of American men are afraid of spiders. More people are afraid of spiders than are afraid of guns, cars or aeroplanes. In a Swedish study of 42 patients with Arachnophobia, it was found that 82 per cent of patients overcame their phobia after just one three-hour therapeutic session where exposure and modelling were used. Those who allegedly suffered or are suffering from this phobia include the great German poet, playwright and historian Johann Christoph Friedrich von Schiller, Esther Rantzen, English actress Wendy Richard, Martina Navratilova, English comedian Phill Jupitus, Johnny Depp, Samantha Fox, US tennis star Andre Agassi, Nell McAndrew, Camilla Dallerup, Ray Park, Justin Timberlake, Nicola McLean and English actor Rupert Grint. Schiller is said to have been so terrified of spiders that if he merely saw one, it made him physically sick.

Case 1: "I'm afraid of spiders. I have always been scared of them. It's not that I can't look at them but the idea of having them touch you or crawling on your body is my greatest fear. Being here in Australia has made me paranoid. The idea of finding one in your bed would just make me want to cry."

Case 2: "I definitely have Arachnophobia, but I can trace its origins to the scar on my abdomen when I was bitten by a black widow. Blech!"[21]

★ ★ ★

ARACHNOPHOBES HAVE "LIMITED INSIGHT" INTO THEIR FEARS
University of Sydney researchers have found that, contrary to prevailing theory, spider phobics "have relatively limited insight into the irrationality of their fears". It is a conventional view in psychiatry that when detached from the phobic situation, people with phobias "can accurately evaluate the danger of potential phobic encounters". They seem to understand how unreasonable their unrealistic fear is and more or less have their fears under control. However, based on

their study of 30 subjects, Drs M.K. Jones and R.G. Menzies found that whether in the presence of the phobic stimulus or not, phobic individuals do not understand their phobias very well at all. Much more public education and community awareness is necessary. [22]

* * *

TOUCH THE SPIDER AND THE FEAR IS MORE LIKELY TO FLEE
A US and Spanish study has discovered that when treating Arachnophobia using virtual reality technology, if the patient is directed to touch the spider during the therapy sessions by touching the computer screen, the therapy becomes twice as effective.[23]

* * *

SPIED UPON (BEING SPIED UPON)
> See Monitored (Being Monitored) — Monitorphobia.

SPIRITS
> See Spectres — Spectrophobia.

SPIRITUAL THINGS
> Pneumatophobia (CP) — From Greek *pneuma* meaning "spirit".

SPLITS
> See Fissures — Fissuraphobia.

SPORTS
> Sports-phobia (SP) — From Latin *sportus* meaning "pass the time". This includes fear of athletic contests. The opposite of this phobia is Sportsophilia, the sexual attraction to sports or athletic contests.

SPORTS UTILITY VEHICLES
> See Cars — Autokinetophobia.

SPORTS UTILITY VEHICLES (BEING A PASSENGER IN A SPORTS UTILITY VEHICLE)

See Cars (Being a Passenger in a Car) — Motorphobia.

SPORTS UTILITY VEHICLES (DRIVING A SPORTS UTILITY VEHICLE)

See Cars (Driving a Car) — Mobilophobia.

SPYING

See Watching — Scopophobia.

STADIUMS

See Theatres — Theatrophobia.

STAGE (THE STAGE)

Topophobia (SP) — From Greek *topos* meaning "a place". This includes fear of acting and performing. Less preferred terms are Ergasiophobia, Ergophobia and Ponophobia. This is sometimes called "stage fright". Among those who suffered from Topophobia in earlier times is the ancient Greek statesman and orator Demosthenes (384–322 BCE), who is described as suffering stage fright by Robert Burton in *The Anatomy of Melancholy*. US actor John Garfield allegedly experienced stage fright. Garfield once confessed: "Yeah, of course [when acting] I get scared. I get scared all the time. When you're up there you might as well be naked! That's scary." English actor, director and producer Laurence Olivier developed Topophobia in the middle of his career. He once wrote: "Stage fright is an animal, a monster which hides in its foul corner without revealing itself, but you know that it is there and that it may come forward at any moment." A contemporary who may suffer from this phobia is English singer and actress Lily Allen. According to one report, "Lily's phobia is getting booed on stage. 'I actually do really believe that people hate me,' she explains, 'and whenever someone introduces me on stage and they go, "Now, Lily Allen," I wait for people to start booing.'"[24]

STAIRS

Climacophobia (TP) — From Greek *klimax* meaning "stair". This includes fear of climbing ramps, climbing stairs, falling down stairs, falling down ramps and ramps. A less preferred term is Bathmophobia.

STAMMERING

See Stuttering — Psellismophobia.

STANDING STILL

Stareophobia (BP) — From Greek *stare* meaning "to stand stiff". Less preferred terms are Ambulophobia, Basiphobia, Stasibasiphobia and Stasiphobia.

STANDING UP

Stasibasiphobia (BP) — From Greek *stasis* meaning "a standing" and *basis* meaning "a step". Less preferred terms are Ambulophobia, Basiphobia, Stareophobia and Stasiphobia. This phobia was once known as Blocq's syndrome after the French physician who first diagnosed it, Paul Oscar Blocq (1860–1896).

STARED AT (BEING STARED AT)

See Monitored (Being Monitored) — Monitorphobia.

STARING

See Watching — Scopophobia.

STARS

Siderophobia (NP) — From Latin *sidero* meaning "star". Less preferred terms are Astraphobia, Astrapophobia, Astrophobia and Astropophobia.

STARVATION

Inanirephobia (BP) — From Latin *inanire* meaning "to make empty or starve". This includes fear of inanition, losing weight and weight loss.

STATUES

Statuophobia (TP) — From Latin *statua* meaning "statue or image". This includes fear of dummies (non-animated human dummies), figurines, mannequins, models and wax models. A less preferred term is Automatonophobia. The opposite of this phobia is Statuophilia, the sexual attraction to statues or mannequins.

STATUS

Timophobia (CP) — From Greek *time* meaning "worth". The opposite of this phobia is Timophilia, the sexual attraction to status or wealth.

STEALING

Kleptophobia (SP) — From Greek *kleptein* meaning "to steal". A less preferred term is Cleptophobia. The opposite of this phobia is Kleptophilia, the sexual attraction to stealing.

STEEP SLOPES

See Cliffs — Cremnophobia.

STEPFATHERS

Vitricophobia (SP) — From Latin *vetrico* meaning "stepfather".

STEPMOTHERS

Novercaphobia (SP) — From Latin *novercalis* meaning "stepmother".

STICKS

See Beaten in Private (Being Beaten in Private) — Rhabdophobia.

STILLNESS

See Alone (Being Alone) — Eremophobia.

STINGERS

Cnidophobia (NP) — From Greek *knide* meaning "stinger". This includes fear of stinging (being stung).

STINGING (BEING STUNG)

See Stingers — Cnidophobia.

STOMACH GURGLING

Borborygamiphobia (BP) — From a modern term, "borborygami" is onomatopoeic. This includes fear of stomach rumbling. Borborygami is the medical term for stomach gurgling or rumbling.

STOMACH RUMBLING

See Stomach Gurgling — Borborygamiphobia.

STOMACH UPSET

Turistaphobia (BP) — From Greek *turisto* meaning "stomach upset".

STOOPING

Kyphophobia (BP) — From Greek *kypho* meaning "stooped or hunchbacked".

STORIES

See Myths — Mythophobia.

STRANGERS

See Foreigners — Xenophobia.

STRANGLING

See Choking (Being Choked) — Pnigophobia.

STREETS

Dromophobia (TP) — From Greek *dromos* meaning "a public way". This includes fear of crossing a street. Less preferred terms are Agoraphobia, Agyiophobia, Agyrophobia and Motorphobia.

STRESS

Strictuphobia (BP) — From Latin *strictus* meaning "strain, compress or draw tight".

STRING

Linonophobia (TP) — From Greek *lino* meaning "cord or thread".

STRIP SHOWS

See Strippers — Ecdysiaphobia.

STRIPPERS

Ecdysiaphobia (SP) — From Greek *ekdusis* meaning "a stripping off". This includes fear of strip shows and striptease.

STRIPTEASE

See Strippers — Ecdysiaphobia.

STROKE

Plegephobia (BP) — From Greek *plege* meaning "stroke".

STUTTERING

Psellismophobia (SP) — From Greek *psellos* meaning "stuttering or stammering". This includes fear of stammering. A less preferred term is Laliophobia.

SUBWAYS

Bathysiderodromophobia (TP) — From Greek *bathys* meaning "deep", *sideros* meaning "iron" and *dromos* meaning "running". This includes fear of underground trains.

SUCCESS

Polycratiphobia (CP) — From Greek *poly* meaning "many" and *kratia* meaning "rule". This includes fear of short-lived success. A less preferred term is Meteorophobia.[25]

SUFFERING

Pathophobia (BP) — From Greek *patho* meaning "disease and suffering". A less preferred term is Panthophobia.

SUFFOCATING

See Choking (Being Choked) — Pnigophobia.

SUICIDE

Suicide-phobia (BP) — From Latin *suicidium* meaning "suicide".

SUN (THE SUN)

Heliophobia (NP) — From Greek *helios* meaning "the sun". This includes fear of radiation (sun's). Less preferred terms are Phegophobia, Phengophobia and Photophobia.

SUNLIGHT

See Daylight — Phengophobia.

SUNSHINE

See Daylight — Phengophobia.

SUPERNATURAL (THE SUPERNATURAL)

Supernaturaphobia (CP) — From Latin *super* meaning "above" and *natura* meaning "nature".

SUPERSTITIONS

Superstitiophobia (CP) — From Latin *superstitionem* meaning "prophecy, soothsaying or excessive fear of the gods".

SURGEONS

See Surgery — Tomophobia.

SURGERY

Tomophobia (BP) — From Greek *tomos* meaning "a slice". This includes fear of surgeons and surgical incisions. Less preferred terms are Ergasiophobia and Ergophobia.

SURGICAL INCISIONS

See Surgery — Tomophobia.

SURVEILLANCE (BEING UNDER SURVEILLANCE)

See Monitored (Being Monitored) — Monitorphobia.

SURVEILLANCING

See Watching — Scopophobia.

SURVEYED (BEING SURVEYED)

See Monitored (Being Monitored) — Monitorphobia.

SURVEYING

See Watching — Scopophobia.

SWALLOWING

See Eating Uncontrollably — Phagophobia.

SWAMPS

See Lakes — Limnophobia.

SWEATING

See Body Fluids — Hygrophobia.

SWEETNESS

Suavisiphobia (NP) — From Latin *suavis* meaning "sweet".

SWIMMING

See Drowning — Aquaphobia.

SWIMMING POOLS

Natatoraphobia (TP) — From Latin *natator* meaning "swimmer". Swimming pools were once called natatoriums. Among those supposedly suffering from this phobia is Christina Ricci, who is "not so keen on swimming pools: 'I won't swim in a pool by myself because I think that somehow a little magic door is going to open up and let the shark out'".[26]

SWORDS

See Pointed Objects — Aichmophobia.

SYMBOLISM
See Symbols — Symbolophobia.

SYMBOLS
Symbolophobia (CP) — From Greek *symbolon* meaning "a token". This includes fear of symbolism.

SYMMETRY
Symmetrophobia (NP) — From Greek *symmetros* meaning "symmetry".

SYPHILIS
Syphilophobia (BP) — From Latin *Syphilus* meaning "plague". Syphilis is a character in a Latin poem by Girolamo Fracastoro (1478–1553), who is infected with the sexually transmitted disease. Lues was the previous name for syphilis. Less preferred terms are Luesophobia and Syphiliphobia.

SYRINGES
See Injections — Trypanophobia.

Chapter 17
Phobias Starting with T

"Fear makes the wolf bigger than he is."
German proverb

TACHYCARDIA

See **Heart Disease** — Cardiopathophobia.

TALKING

See **Speaking** — Phonophobia.

TALKING WHILE EATING

See **Dining** — Deipnophobia.

TALL BUILDINGS

See **High Buildings** — Batophobia.

TALL OBJECTS

See **High Buildings** — Batophobia.

TAOISM

Taoisiophobia (CP) — From Chinese *tao* meaning "the way, the path, the right way of life". It can refer to fear of Taoist doctrine, gatherings, people, rituals or anything else Taoist.

TAPEWORMS

Taeniophobia (AP) — From Latin *taenia* meaning "ribbon". Less preferred terms are Taeniphobia, Teniophobia and Teniphobia.

Case: A 27-year-old woman says that she has been afraid of tapeworms since she had to examine one in a biology class in high school. "It was horrible. I imagine this awful thing living inside of my stomach. It makes me want to drink acid to kill it. I cook all the meat I eat until it is almost black. I want to kill off any chance of being infected with a tapeworm. My little sister had worms when she was about eight or nine. I was terrified I would get them too, but didn't somehow. I still fear I will have tapeworms living inside of me if I'm not careful. I'm afraid that one will crawl up through my throat and come out my mouth. There is nothing more disgusting."

TASTE

Geumaphobia (BP) — From Greek *geume* meaning "taste". Less preferred terms are Geumatophobia and Geumophobia.

TATTOOS

Tattoo-phobia (TP) — From Polynesian *tattoo* meaning "mark the skin with pigment".

TEARS

Dacryphobia (BP) — From Greek *dacryon* meaning "tear". The opposite of this phobia is Dacryphilia, the sexual attraction to tears.

TECHNOLOGY

Technophobia (TP) — From Greek *techne* meaning "art, craft or skill".

TEDDY BEARS

Archtophobia (TP) — From Greek *arkhos* meaning "chief or leader". This is a reference to US President Theodore Roosevelt, after whom the first teddy bear was named in 1903.

TEENAGERS

Hebephobia (SP) — From Greek *hebe* meaning "youthfulness". A less preferred term is Ephebiphobia. The opposite of this phobia is Hebephilia, the sexual attraction to teenagers.

TEETH

Odontophobia (BP) — From Greek *odontos* meaning "tooth". The opposite of this phobia is Odontophilia, the sexual attraction to teeth or the mouth of a sexual partner.

Case: "I'm a male in my early 60s. Since a boy I've had this strange fear of my teeth falling out of my jaw, especially when I'm sleeping. This really happened to me twice when I was losing teeth as a child. I was sleeping on my back and I woke up feeling a tooth rolling around in my mouth. One had come loose and fallen out. A few months later I woke up with one tooth missing. I must have swallowed it as I was sleeping during the night. I searched around my bed but couldn't find it. This annoyed me no end at the time because the Tooth Fairy gave me a coin for each tooth I lost. Since then every time my teeth or gums feel sensitive, I get fearful. Sometimes I can't sleep."

TELEPHONES

Telephonophobia (TP) — From a modern term, "telephone" is derived from Greek *telos* meaning "end" and *phonetikos* meaning "vocal". This includes fear of speaking on the telephone. A less preferred term is Phonophobia. English actress Helen Mirren supposedly experiences tremendous fear when merely thinking of talking on the telephone. According to one report, David Gest also suffers from this phobia.[1]

TELEVISION

TV-phobia (TP) — From a modern term, "TV" is short for "television". If you are a TV-phobe, you share this with US actress

Sharon Stone, who supposedly "does not switch on the TV if she is alone in a room. It seems to her that it can blow up every minute."[2]

TEMPOROMANDIBULAR JOINT DISORDER

TMJ-phobia (BP) — From Latin *tempora* meaning "side of the forehead" and *manibula* meaning "jaw". "TMJ" is an acronym for the medical condition of temporomandibular joint disorder. TMJ is an umbrella term covering acute, chronic and often very painful inflammation of the temporomandibular joint connecting the jaw with the skull.

TERMINOLOGY

See Scientific Terms — Hellenologophobia.

TERMITES

Isopterophobia (AP) — From Greek *iso* meaning "termite". This includes fear of white ants and wood-eating insects.

TERRAPINS

See Turtles — Chelonaphobia.

TERROR

See Fears — Phobophobia.

TERRORISM

Terror-phobia (SP) — From Latin *terrorem* meaning "great fear". This includes fear of terrorists. Terrorism has emerged as a common fear in our post-9/11 world. However, your chance of dying via an act of terrorism is less than your chance of dying by choking on a peanut.

Case: A 45-year-old woman says, "I no longer go to Bali after the bombing of a nightclub there ten years ago. A terrorist bomb freaks me. They could be anywhere. When I walk by a rubbish bin in the middle of Sydney, I wonder if a bomb may be hidden inside. Whenever I board a plane, I wonder if there's a bomb on board too."

TERRORISTS

See Terrorism — Terror-phobia.

TESTS (ACADEMIC)

See Examinations (Academic) — Examinaphobia.

TESTS (NON-ACADEMIC)

See Social Situations — Sociophobia.

TETANUS

Tetanophobia (BP) — From Greek *tetanois* meaning "muscle spasm or tension". Tetanus (also known as lockjaw) is a medical condition characterised by prolonged contraction of skeletal muscle fibres.

TEXTURES (CERTAIN TEXTURES)

Textophobia (NP) — From Latin *textere* meaning "to weave".

THEATRES

Theatrophobia (TP) — From Greek *theatron* meaning "a theatre". This includes fear of auditoriums, classrooms and stadiums.

THEOLOGY

Theologicophobia (CP) — From Greek *theo* meaning "god".

THIEVES

See Bad People — Scelerophobia.

THINKING (IRRATIONAL)

Aphronemophobia (BP) — From Greek *a* meaning "away from" and *phront* meaning "thought or attention". This includes fear of irrationality and thought (irrational).

THINKING (RATIONAL)

Phronemophobia (BP) — From Greek *phroneein* meaning "to think". This includes fear of meditation and thought (rational).

A less preferred term is Phrenophobia. Philosopher Bertrand Russell (1872–1970) once wrote: "Men fear thought as they fear nothing else on earth — more than ruin, more even than death."

THIRTEEN (NUMBER 13)

Triskaidekaphobia (CP) — From Greek *tris* meaning "three", *kai* meaning "and" and *deka* meaning "ten". Less preferred terms are Terdekaphobia, Tredecaphobia and Tridecaphobia. Thirty-second US President Franklin Roosevelt allegedly suffered from this phobia. One of the most famous quotes about fear is Roosevelt's. It is part of his first inaugural address given on 4 March 1933 in the midst of the Great Depression of the 1930s: "The only thing we have to fear is fear itself — nameless, unreasoning, unjustified terror which paralyses needed efforts to convert retreat into advance." Diana, Princess of Wales, also supposedly experienced this phobia and this was respected even after her death. The auction of evening dresses that she wore just before her death did not include a catalogued Number 13; the auction jumped from Number 12 to Number 14.[3]

THOUGHT (IRRATIONAL)

See **Thinking (Irrational)** — Aphronemophobia.

THOUGHT (RATIONAL)

See **Thinking (Rational)** — Phronemophobia.

THRESHOLDS

Bathmophobia (TP) — From Greek *bathmos* meaning "a step of high depth". This includes fear of crossing a threshold.[4]

THROWN OBJECTS

See **Bullets** — Ballistophobia.

THUNDER

Brontophobia (NP) — From Greek *bronto* meaning "thunder".

This includes fear of thunderbolts and thunderstorms. Less preferred terms are Astraphobia, Astrapophobia, Astrophobia, Astropophobia, Ceraunophobia, Ceraynophobia, Keraunophobia, Keuranosophobia and Tonitrophobia. Among those who suffered or are suffering from this phobia are James Joyce and US singer and actress Madonna. One biographer writes of Joyce: "He also suffered from a fear of thunderstorms, which his deeply religious aunt had described to him as being a sign of God's wrath. Asked why he was afraid of thunder when his children weren't, 'Ah,' said Joyce in contempt, 'they have no religion'. His fears were part of his identity, and he had no wish, even if he had had the power, to slough any of them off."

Case: A 61-year-old woman says, "I am terrified of thunder and have been from as early as I can remember. I remember being at school as a little girl. A thunderstorm shook the schoolroom. The windows rattled and our teacher was terrified. I fear a sonic boom too. It is like thunder. I no longer hide in a closet when I hear thunder, but I used to."[5]

THUNDERBOLTS

See Thunder — Brontophobia.

THUNDERSTORMS

See Thunder — Brontophobia.

TICKLED (BEING TICKLED)

Titillarephobia (SP) — From Latin *titillare* meaning "to touch lightly so as to cause a peculiar or uneasy sensation". A less preferred term is Pteronophobia.

Case: "This one is very odd and I'm sure no one else has this except me. I have a phobia of being tickled. All my life it's been this way for me. If I'm tickled, I think I will run out of air and suffocate. How's that for a strange one!"

TIDAL WAVES

See Earthquakes — Seismosophobia.

TIDINESS

Taxophobia (CP) — From Greek *taxo* meaning "order".

TIED UP (BEING TIED UP)

See Bound (Being Bound) — Merinthophobia.

TIGERS

Tigrisophobia (AP) — From Latin *tigris* meaning "tiger".

TIME

Chronophobia (NP) — From Greek *chronos* meaning "age". This includes fear of age differences, deadlines, duration of an event, schedules and timetables. The opposite of this phobia is Chronophilia, the sexual attraction to someone of a great age difference.

TIME (TRAVELLING BACK IN TIME)

Retrotempophobia (CP) — From Latin *retro* meaning "backward" and *tempus* meaning "time". No one has been able to do it, but that has not stopped some people from being afraid of it.

TIMETABLES

See Time — Chronophobia.

TOADS

Bufonophobia (AP) — From Latin *bufonidae* meaning "true toads". Less preferred terms are Batrachophobia and Ranidaphobia.

TOBACCO

See Smoking — Smykheinophobia.

TOENAILS

See Nails (Fingers or Toes) — Onychophobia.

TOILETS (PRIVATE)

See Washing — Ablutophobia.

TOILETS (PUBLIC)

See Lavatories — Lavatoriphobia.

TOMBS

See Cemeteries — Coimetrophobia.

TOMBSTONES

Placophobia (TP) — From Latin *placi* meaning "calm or peace".

TONGUES

See Public Speaking — Glossophobia.

TOOTHACHES

Odontoachophobia (BP) — From Greek *odontos* meaning "tooth" and *akhos* meaning "pain or distress".

TORNADOES

See Violent Storms — Lilapsophobia.

TORTOISES

See Turtles — Chelonaphobia.

TORTURE (BEING TORTURED)

See Pain (One's Own) — Algophobia.

TOUCHED (BEING TOUCHED)

Haphephobia (SP) — From Greek *haphe* meaning "touch". This includes fear of massages (being massaged). Less preferred terms are Aphenphosmphobia, Aphephobia, Chiraptophobia, Haptephobia, Haptophobia and Thixophobia. English–Canadian actor and comedian Mike Myers and English actress, model, fashion designer and singer Kelly Osbourne have an aversion to being touched. According to one report, Osbourne is particularly afraid of her collarbone being touched.[6]

TOUCHING (TOUCHING OBJECTS OR THINGS)

Tangerephobia (BP) — From Latin *tangere* meaning "to touch".

TOUCHING (TOUCHING PEOPLE)

Sarmassophobia (SP) — From Greek *sarx* meaning "flesh" and *massein* meaning "to touch or knead". The opposite of this phobia is Sarmassophilia, the sexual attraction to touching.

TOURETTE'S SYNDROME

See Autism — Autism-phobia.

TRAINS

Siderodromophobia (TP) — From Greek *sideros* meaning "iron" and *dromos* meaning "running". This includes fear of railway lines, railway tracks and railways. A less preferred term is Sideromophobia. The opposite of this phobia is Siderodromophilia, the sexual attraction to trains. Sigmund Freud allegedly suffered from Siderodromophobia. According to one account, this phobia originated in Freud's childhood when during "a trip from Freiberg [Germany] the train passed through Breslau, where Freud saw gas jets for the first time; they made him think of souls burning in hell".[7]

TRAMPS

See Beggars — Mendicarephobia.

TRANQUILLISERS

See Medicines — Pharmacophobia.

TRAUMA

Traumatophobia (BP) — From Greek *trauma* meaning "a wound". This includes fear of injury and wounds.

TRAVEL

Hodophobia (BP) — From Greek *hodos* meaning "way or path".
This includes fear of road travel. The opposite of this phobia
is Hodophilia, the sexual attraction to travel. Sigmund Freud
allegedly suffered from Hodophobia and was terrified of train
travel in particular.

Case 1: "[When I travel] I am afraid of parking ramps; yes, that's
right, parking ramps. It just is unbelievable to me that a bunch of
concrete and such can hold up that much weight. I start looking
at the structure and think it will collapse on me or something.
Coming out of them is the worst, especially when it is one of those
tight windy twisty columns and there is a ton of people in line. I
just freak out and start having a panic attack. I am curious if there
is a name for this phobia."

Case 2: "… the freeways in LA. I came from a small town and
we didn't have any of the huge highway systems like LA does.
When I moved out to LA and saw on the news some photos of
all of the mangled cars in a huge pile-up, it scared the hell out of
me. Sometimes I zone out when I'm on the freeway and I can just
imagine the car I am in getting into one of those accidents. The
thought of how fast everyone behind you is going, and that they
may not be able to stop and that they could just cause a massive
number of cars to all mush together! Who wouldn't be scared of
that?"[8]

TREES

Dendrophobia (NP) — From Greek *dendron* meaning "a tree". The
opposite of this phobia is Dendrophilia, the sexual attraction to
trees.

TREMBLING

Tremophobia (BP) — From Latin *tremere* meaning "to shake". This
includes fear of shaking and tremors.

TREMORS

See **Trembling** — Tremophobia.

TRICHINOSIS

Trichinophobia (BP) — From Greek *trikhos* meaning "hair-like". Trichinosis is a medical condition caused by a hair-like parasitic roundworm, known as the trichina worm, which is transmitted to humans by eating raw or undercooked pig.

TRUCKS

See **Cars** — Autokinetophobia.

TRUCKS (BEING A PASSENGER IN A TRUCK)

See **Cars (Being a Passenger in a Car)** — Motorphobia.

TRUCKS (DRIVING A TRUCK)

See **Cars (Driving a Car)** — Mobilophobia.

TSUNAMI

See **Earthquakes** — Seismosophobia.

TUBERCULOSIS

Tuberculophobia (BP) — From Latin *tuberculum* meaning "a little tube". A less preferred term is Phthisiophobia. Tuberculosis (TB) is a medical condition caused by a bacterial infection affecting the lungs and other parts of the body.

TUBES

See **Tunnels** — Tubuphobia.

TUNNELS

Tubuphobia (TP) — From Latin *tubus* meaning "tube, pipe or tunnel". This includes fear of pipes (hollow) and tubes. Woody Allen and Matthew McConaughey are allegedly terrified of tunnels.[9]

TURTLES

Chelonaphobia (AP) — From Greek *chelone* meaning "turtle".
This includes fear of terrapins and tortoises. According to one
report, a primary school teacher in Sheldon, Iowa, helped children
overcome their "natural" Chelonaphobia by having each child care
for a turtle and enter it in a turtle race. Too bad all phobias are not
eliminated when we are in primary school and by entering them in
a race.[10]

TWINS

Biniphobia (SP) — From Latin *bini* meaning "two each".

TYPHOONS

See Violent Storms — Lilapsophobia.

TYRANTS

Tyranophobia (SP) — From Greek *tyrannus* meaning "a tyrant".
A less preferred term is Tyrannophobia.

Chapter 18
Phobias Starting with U & V

"In politics, what begins in fear usually ends in folly."

Samuel Taylor Coleridge (1772–1834), *Specimens of the Table Talk*

U (LETTER)

U-phobia (CP) — From the Greek letter *U* and the 21st letter of the English alphabet.

Case: "The letter U is frightening to me. It has been since I was in school. I imagine myself falling from the two tops of the letter down into the bottom, where I cannot climb out. It is like I have been swallowed. I know it is silly, but I can't bear to look at a U. And the name of the letter frightens me too. 'U' means 'you'. It is as if the letter U is following me. When it catches up it will swallow me. I know it is silly, silly."

UFOs

UFO-phobia (TP) — From modern terms, "UFO" is an acronym for unidentified flying object. Many such UFOs are natural phenomena while others are of human invention.

Case: A 26-year-old woman says, "I believe in UFOs. I know it's crazy. I feel like a dill in telling you. I'm afraid that one of them will swoop down some night and take me away, rape me and probably dissect my body too. I've told one or two friends and they think I'm so weird."

UGLINESS

Cacophobia (CP) — From Greek *kako* meaning "bad or evil".
A less preferred term is Teratophobia.

UGLY PEOPLE

See Deformity — Dysmorphophobia.

ULCERS

Ulcerisiophobia (BP) — From Latin *ulceris* meaning "ulcer".

UNCLEANLINESS

Rhypophobia (NP) — From Greek *rhyparos* meaning "dirty". This
includes fear of contamination, dirt and filth. Less preferred terms
are Automysophobia, Coprophobia, Misophobia, Molysmophobia,
Molysomophobia, Mysophobia, Rupophobia, Rypophobia,
Scatophobia, Spermophobia and Verminophobia. Woody Allen
is terrified of dirty water; he will not take baths, only showers.
When Allen was in a relationship with US actress Mia Farrow and
stayed at her country home for the first time, he had to return to
New York because the house had no shower. A shower was then
constructed just for him. US model and actress Kim Kardashian is
supposedly obsessively afraid that her ears will become dirty. She
cleans them with cotton swabs five times per day. US actress and
singer Hilary Duff is allegedly so frightened of dirt that she cannot
go to bed until she cleans the bedroom. Scarlett Johansson is
reportedly so fearful of dirt that she prefers to clean her hotel room
herself long before a maid arrives to perform this task.

Case: A 57-year-old woman says, "I fear dirt. If a spot is on my
clothes I have to change immediately. And I mean immediately. I
hate filth, rubbish and germs. I wish I could stay in the bath all day.
It is the only place where I know I will stay clean. My mother used
to use disinfectant on me. I love the smell of disinfectant because it
is the smell of being clean."[1]

UNCONSCIOUSNESS
Aconsciusiophobia (BP) — From Latin *a* meaning "not" and *conscius* meaning "knowing or aware".

UNDERGROUND TRAINS
See Subways — Bathysiderodromophobia.

UNDERWEAR
See Lingerie — Lingeriephobia.

UNDRESSING
Dishabiliophobia (SP) — From Greek *adysois* meaning "undress" and *habili* meaning "clothing".

Case: "I hate to undress in front of people. I hated to do this in PE classes in school. I avoided swimming in school too whenever I could. I made all sorts of excuses. I always tried to get as far away from others as possible when I had to undress. I am afraid of undressing in front of a doctor. I hate medical exams. It is a little easier in front of another woman so I always have a woman doctor. I even have trouble undressing in front of my husband. I guess it is my Catholic girlhood."

UNFAMILIAR (THE UNFAMILIAR)
See New (Anything New) — Neophobia.

UNIFORMS
Uniformophobia (TP) — From Latin *unus* meaning "one or same" and *forma* meaning "form". The opposite of this phobia is Uniformophilia, the sexual attraction to a partner dressed in a uniform or special clothing.

UNKNOWN (THE UNKNOWN)
Agnosophobia (BP) — From Greek *a* meaning "not" and *gno* meaning "know".

UNMARRIED (BEING UNMARRIED)

Anuptaphobia (SP) — From Greek *anupta* meaning "growing old alone". This includes fear of single (being single).

UNORTHODOXY

See Heresy — Hereiophobia.

UNPRONOUNCEABLE WORDS

See Words (Long or Unpronounceable) — Sesquipedalophobia.

UNTIDINESS

See Disorder — Ataxiophobia.

URINARY INCONTINENCE

Incontinephobia (BP) — From Latin *incontinentem* meaning "not containing". This includes fear of incontinence. Incontinence is a medical condition characterised by an involuntary loss of bladder or bowel control.

Case: "I'm afraid that I will be somewhere where I can't find a toilet. Whenever I plan wherever I will go, I always think about where the toilets will be. I have a very small bladder. I will go to the toilet sometimes 10 times a day. Sometimes I go to the toilet even when I don't have to. I always make sure my bladder is empty before I go out of the house. I want to make sure I won't need a toilet. But if I do, I'll know where one is."

URINE

Urophobia (BP) — From Latin *urina* meaning "urine". A less preferred term is Urinophobia. The opposite of this phobia is Urophilia, the sexual attraction to behaviours involving urine.

USING THE WRONG WORDS

See Speaking — Phonophobia.

VACCINATIONS

Vaccinophobia (TP) — From Latin *vaccinus* meaning "from a cow". This includes fear of inoculations. A less preferred term is Trypanophobia. Physician Edward Jenner (1749–1823) prevented humans contracting the more dangerous smallpox virus by inoculating them with the less dangerous cowpox virus.

VACUUMS

See Barren Spaces — Kenophobia.

VAGINAS

Eurotophobia (BP) — From Greek *eu* meaning "well" and *eurythmos* meaning "wide and rhythmical". This includes fear of female genitals and genitals (female). Less preferred terms are Colpophobia, Eurotrophobia and Kolpophobia.

VAGRANTS

See Beggars — Mendicarephobia.

VAMPIRES

Lemurephobia (CP) — From Latin *lemurs* meaning "spirits of the dead".

Case: An 18-year-old male says, "When I was a kid I used to be super-freaked out by vampires. I was afraid they'd come in the night and suck out my blood. I'm not so bad any more."

VEGETABLES

Lachanophobia (NP) — From Greek *lachan* meaning "vegetable".

VEHICLES

See Cars — Autokinetophobia.

VEHICLES (BEING A PASSENGER IN A VEHICLE)

See Cars (Being a Passenger in a Car) — Motorphobia.

VEHICLES (DRIVING A VEHICLE)

See Cars (Driving a Car) — Mobilophobia.

VENEREAL DISEASES

See Sexually Transmitted Diseases — Cypriphobia.

VENTRILOQUISTS

Ventriloquaphobia (TP) — From Latin *venter* meaning "belly" and *loqui* meaning "speak". A less preferred term is Automatonophobia.

VERBAL SLIPS

See Speaking — Phonophobia.

VERMIN

Vermiphobia (AP) — From Latin *vermis* meaning "a worm".

VERTIGO

See Dizziness — Illyngophobia.

VESSELS

See Ships — Nautophobia.

VIOLENCE

Violentiaphobia (SP) — From Latin *violentia* meaning "violence". This includes fear of random violence and workplace violence.

VIOLENT STORMS

Lilapsophobia (NP) — From Greek *lilapso* meaning "violent storm". This includes fear of hurricanes, tornadoes and typhoons.

VIRGINITY

Eisodophobia (BP) — From Greek *eisodo* meaning "way within". Less preferred terms are Esodophobia, Lysuseisodophobia and Primeisodophobia.

VIRGINS

See Girls — Parthenophobia.

VOICE (ANOTHER'S)

Voxiphobia (SP) — From Latin *vox* meaning "voice, sound, utterance, cry or call". This includes fear of loud talking, murmuring, shouting, singing, soft talking, whispering and whistling. Less preferred terms are Acousticophobia and Phonophobia.

VOICE (ONE'S OWN)

See Speaking — Phonophobia.

VOIDS

See Barren Spaces — Kenophobia.

VOMIT (ANOTHER'S)

See Vomiting — Emetophobia.

VOMIT (ONE'S OWN)

See Vomiting — Emetophobia.

VOMITING

Emetophobia (BP) — From Greek *emetikos* meaning "vomit". This includes fear of saliva, vomit (another's) and vomit (one's own). The opposite of this phobia is Emetophilia, the sexual attraction to vomit or vomiting. If you are an Emetophobe, you share this with famed US singer, songwriter and social activist Joan Baez, US TV presenter Matt Lauer, US model and actress Denise Richards, and English writer and TV presenter Charlie Brooker.

Case: A 19-year-old male says, "I have a fear of vomit. My own or somebody else's. The thought of it makes me want to vomit. I remember stepping in some vomit at school when another kid was sick. For years after that I kept checking my shoes every night to make sure I hadn't stepped on that vomit again. I'd better stop talking about it now."

VOMITING DUE TO AIR SICKNESS

See Air Sickness — Aeronausiphobia.

VOODOO

Voodoophobia (CP) — From Haitian *vodu* meaning "spirit, demon or deity".

VOYEURING

See Watching — Scopophobia.

Chapter 19
Phobias Starting with
W, X, Y & Z

"Fear is more pain than is the pain it fears."
Sir Philip Sidney (1554–1586), *Arcadia*

WAITING

Macrophobia (SP) — From Greek *macro* meaning "long or large". This includes fear of long waits. Mental health professionals have been using this term for years. We have the Greek "long", but where is the Greek "wait" in this term? It seems we will have to wait for an explanation. Hope we do not have to wait too long — especially Macrophobes.

WALKING

Basiophobia (BP) — From Greek *basis* meaning "a step". This includes fear of falling and mobility. Less preferred terms are Ambulophobia, Baraphobia, Barophobia, Basiphobia, Basistasiphobia, Basophobia, Basostasophobia, Stasibasiphobia, Stasiphobia and Stasophobia.

★ ★ ★

THE ETHNIC FACTOR IN PHOBIAS
Ethnicity is often a factor in phobias. We humans see the world through many lenses. One of these is culture. How a culture shapes our vision

of reality shows itself in numerous ways, including through phobias. An example of this is the strange finding that African-Americans have unusually high rates of Basiophobia, especially as it relates to falling. Fear of falling, once believed to be mostly a problem for senior citizens, in fact strikes African-American middle-aged adults in disproportionate numbers and with negative consequences to their health. According to Dr Margaret Mary Wilson, "African-American middle-aged adults, some as young as 50, say they are so afraid of falling that they become less active, which creates a cycle that causes frailty and illness. Among middle-aged African-Americans, there's this huge fear of falling, which many of us thought existed only in older adults. This is strange because this fear of falling exists in people who have never fallen before. It's an illogical fear. Yet they're so afraid of falling that they avoid activities. It becomes a self-fulfilling prophecy. They become weak and they fall." Dr Wilson adds that "falling was surprisingly high among middle-aged African-Americans who live in the inner city. About one in three people feared falling, making the fear as common among these middle-aged adults as it is among the elderly." Dr Wilson led a study of nearly 1,000 African-American subjects living in both poor and affluent communities.[1]

* * *

WALLOON (THINGS WALLOON)

Walloonphobia (CP) — A modern term, "Walloon" is a derivation of *Wallon* meaning "foreigner".

WAR

Bellumaphobia (SP) — From Latin *bellum* meaning "conflict, strife or struggle".

WASHING

Ablutophobia (BP) — From Latin *ablutio* meaning "wash away". This includes fear of bathing (washing), bathrooms (private bathrooms) and toilets (private toilets). The opposite of this phobia is Ablutophilia, the sexual attraction to washing with water.

Frederick the Great of Prussia was so fearful of washing and water that he could not wash himself with water. Instead, his servants had to wipe him down with dry towels.

Case: "I have ... problems with going into a restroom that has a shower with the curtain closed. I have to open it before I can do anything."[2]

WASPS

Spheksophobia (AP) — From Greek *spheka* meaning "a wasp". English actor, singer, songwriter and TV presenter Robson Green allegedly experiences this phobia.[3]

WATCHING

Scopophobia (SP) — From Greek *scopo* meaning "examine". This includes fear of bugging, looking, scrutinising, seeing, spying, staring, surveillancing, surveying and voyeuring. Less preferred terms are Ophthalmophobia and Scoptophobia. The opposite of this phobia is Scopophilia, the sexual attraction to watching sexual activity (voyeurism).

WATER

Hydrophobia (NP) — From Greek *hydro* meaning "water". This includes fear of dampness, humidity, liquids, moisture and wetness. Less preferred terms are Aquaphobia, Equaphobia, Hydrophobophobia, Hygrophobia, Nautophobia and Potamophobia. Those who allegedly suffered or are suffering from this phobia include Frederick the Great, Shemp Howard, Esther Rantzen and English actress Joanna Lumley.[4]

WATERFALLS

Casicarephobia (NP) — From Latin *casicare* meaning "to fall". Among those who allegedly suffer from this phobia is David Boreanaz. As he explained, "You just want to jump into a waterfall, they are really scary."

Case 1: A 58-year-old man says, "I'm not keen on waterfalls. When I toured the American national parks as a youth I got alongside the top of a waterfall that had a very deep drop. I was told that some people wandered into the stream (or river), got caught in the current and went over the falls. I had nightmares about this for years. I guess I'm afraid of heights too, but especially of waterfalls."

Case 2: "I am completely afraid of waterfalls. I'm not sure whether it's the sight of that huge volume of water crashing on the rocks or the sound that is worse. The two together make it impossible for me to visit any places with waterfalls or even look at them on TV. We went to Yosemite two months ago and I spent almost the whole trip with my eyes and ears shut! A trip to Niagara or Victoria Falls would be the most frightening thing I could ever do — even saying 'Niagara' makes me shiver down my spine! Nothing to do with heights ... I could stand on the edge of the Grand Canyon, no prob. And I have no issue with lakes, although man-made dams make me feel uneasy."[5]

WAVE-LIKE MOTIONS

See Waves — Kymophobia.

WAVES

Kymophobia (NP) — From Greek *kymo* meaning "wave". This includes fear of wave-like motions. A less preferred term is Cymophobia.

WAX MODELS

See Statues — Statuophobia.

WEAKNESS

Asthenophobia (BP) — From Greek *a* meaning "without" and *sthenos* meaning "strength". This includes fear of collapsing and fainting. Less preferred terms are Ashenophobia and

Basostasophobia. Weakness, collapsing or fainting can be the phobic stimulus and also a reaction to a phobia. When US researchers gave surveys to 934 fainters and non-fainters to find out in which medical situation people were most afraid, it was found that 72 per cent of fainters and 47 per cent of non-fainters thought that "fear of injections and blood draws" was the most frightening.[6]

WEALTH

Plutophobia (CP) — From Greek *pluto* meaning "wealth". Less preferred terms are Aurophobia and Chrematophobia. Pluto was the Greek god of wealth.

WEASELS

Galeophobia (AP) — From Greek *galeos* meaning "cat-like". This includes fear of badgers, ferrets, polecats and raccoons.

Case 1: "I have a great phobia of raccoons. I immediately start sobbing uncontrollably [when I see one]. I can't look at one or see one crossing the street. I even get panic attacks."

Case 2: "I also have a phobia of raccoons. If I'm walking and I see one on the sidewalk or in the street, I get an immediate panic attack and just run. This has almost gotten me hit by two cars. If I still see it [the raccoon] coming in my direction, I just start crying."

Case 3: "Call me strange if you want. I know the ferrets are cute and all … to you. I see them as creepy little nocturnal rodents with evil teeth that will fly out of the night sky and nibble on your toes. Shivers!"[7]

WEDDINGS

See Ceremonies — Teleophobia.

WEIGHT DIFFERENCES

Veherevahtophobia (NP) — From Greek *vehereva* meaning "heavy or light". The opposite of this phobia is Veherevahtophilia, the sexual attraction to a great weight difference in a sexual partner.

WEIGHT GAIN

See Obesity — Obesophobia.

WEIGHT LOSS

See Starvation — Inanirephobia.

WEREWOLVES

See Wolves — Lycanthropophobia.

WET DREAMS

Oneirogmophobia (BP) — From Greek *oneiro* meaning "to dream".

WETNESS

See Water — Hydrophobia.

WHALES

See Marine Mammals — Cetusaphobia.

WHEAT

Darataphobia (NP) — From Greet *darata* meaning "bread".

WHIPPED (BEING WHIPPED IN PRIVATE)

See Beaten in Private (Being Beaten in Private) — Rhabdophobia.

WHIPPED (BEING WHIPPED IN PUBLIC)

See Beaten in Public (Being Beaten in Public) — Mastigophobia.

WHIRLPOOLS

Dinophobia (NP) — From Greek *dino* meaning "whirlpools or eddies". A less preferred term is Vertigophobia.

WHISPERING

See Voice (Another's) — Voxiphobia.

WHISTLING

See Voice (Another's) — Voxiphobia.

WHITE (COLOUR OR WORD)

Leukophobia (NP) — From Greek *leuko* meaning "white".

WHITE ANTS

See Termites — Isopterophobia.

WICKED PEOPLE

See Bad People — Scelerophobia.

WILD ANIMALS

See Animals (Wild) — Agrizoophobia.

WIND

Anemophobia (NP) — From Greek *anemos* meaning "wind or breath". This includes fear of air draughts, draughts and gales. Less preferred terms are Aerophobia and Ancraophobia.

Case: "I know this is strange but I have a huge fear of walking down the road and the wind all of a sudden blowing my clothes off. I also have a fear of a fish getting out of its tank in the middle of the night and sucking on me till I have no blood left. I also have a fear of dying."[8]

WIND INSTRUMENTS

Aulophobia (TP) — From Greek *aulos* meaning "wind instrument". This includes fear of brass instruments, flutes and woodwind instruments. A less preferred term is Autophobia. One of the earliest accounts of Aulophobia is by the ancient Greek physician Hippocrates. He writes of: "… the morbid condition of Nicanor. When he used to begin drinking, the girl flute-player would frighten him; as soon as he heard the first note of the flute at a banquet, he would be beset by terror. He used to say he could scarcely contain himself when night fell; but during the day he would hear this instrument without feeling any emotion. This lasted a long time with him."[9]

WINE

Oenophobia (TP) — From Greek *oeino* meaning "wine". A less preferred term is Oinophobia.

WINGS

Pennaphobia (NP) — From Latin *penna* meaning "wing".

WISDOM

See Learning — Sophophobia.

WITCHCRAFT

Wiccaphobia (CP) — From Latin *wicca* meaning "pagan". This includes fear of witches.

WITCHES

See Witchcraft — Wiccaphobia.

WOLVERINES

Gulophobia (AP) — From Latin *gulo* meaning "glutton".

WOLVES

Lycanthropophobia (AP) — From Greek *lycos* meaning "wolf". This includes fear of werewolves. Wolves do not rampage throughout Europe the way they used to a few hundred years ago. The number of Lycanthropophobes, like the number of wolves, is small today, but wolf and werewolf fears were very real in the past. The German proverb still rings true: "Fear makes the wolf bigger than he is."[10]

WOMEN

Gynephobia (SP) — From Greek *gyne* meaning "female". This includes fear of females. Less preferred terms are Caligynephobia, Feminophobia, Gynophobia and Venustraphobia. An older and quaint Latin expression for this phobia is *horror feminae* meaning "horrible women".

WOOD

Xylophobia (NP) — From Greek *xylo* meaning "wood". This includes fear of wooden objects. Less preferred terms are Hylephobia and Hylophobia.

WOOD-EATING INSECTS

See Termites — Isopterophobia.

WOODEN OBJECTS

See Wood — Xylophobia.

WOODS (THE WOODS)

See Forests — Hylophobia.

WOODS AT NIGHT

See Forests at Night — Nyctohylophobia.

WOODWIND INSTRUMENTS

See Wind Instruments — Aulophobia.

WORDS

Logophobia (CP) — From Greek *logos* meaning "word". Less preferred terms are Nomatophobia, Nomenatophobia, Onomatophobia and Verbophobia.[11]

WORDS (LONG OR UNPRONOUNCEABLE)

Sesquipedalophobia (CP) — From Latin *sesqui* meaning "one and a half" and *pedalis* meaning "of the foot". It literally means "one and a half feet". This includes fear of long words and unpronounceable words. Less preferred terms are Hellenologophobia, Hippotomonstrosesquippedaliophobia, Macroxenoglossophobia and Sequipedalophobia. These even longer terms may have been an intentional exaggeration to emphasise word length. Ironically, if you suffer from this phobia, you would be afraid of the word for it.

WORK

Ergasiophobia (BP) — From Greek *ergasia* meaning "work". This includes fear of action, functioning, operating and overworking. Less preferred terms are Ergophobia, Kopophobia and Ponophobia.

WORKPLACE VIOLENCE

See Violence — Violentiaphobia.

WORM INFESTATION

See Worms — Helminthophobia.

WORMS

Helminthophobia (AP) — From Greek *helminthos* meaning "worms". This includes fear of worm infestation. Less preferred terms are Scoleciphobia, Taeniphobia, Taeniophobia, Teniophobia, Teniphobia, Verminophobia and Vermiphobia. A caller to the Richard Glover programme on ABC Radio in Sydney said that "for my entire life I have been afraid of worms. It started when I stepped on some when I was young."

Case 1: "I have some very strange fears … for one I am deathly afraid of worms … even spelling it freaks me out … so I refer to them as squigglys … but if I see one I start to freak out … sometimes resulting in me crying for a while."

Case 2: "Whenever it rains [and] worms come out of their holes I get sick to my stomach [and] I can feel them under my feet for days. It grosses [me out and] when it rains you can also smell them. I also have a phobia of caterpillars. It's pretty much the same as the worms but worse. The thought of them sends shivers up my spine."

Case 3: "[I have an] intense phobia of nails, lugs and orms. So much so that I don't even want to type out the full words. My significant other (and almost everyone else, really) thinks it's hilariously absurd. I mean, snakes, sharks and spiders can bite and potentially kill you, and they're quick. S.O. poking fun at me: 'Aaaaahhhhh, run faster! They're gaining on you!'"[12]

WOUNDS
See Trauma — Traumatophobia.

WRINKLES
Rhytiphobia (BP) — From Greek *rhytis* meaning "a wrinkle".

WRITING
See Handwriting — Graphophobia.

WRITING IN PUBLIC
See Handwriting in Public — Scriptophobia.

WRONGDOINGS
See Errors — Hamartophobia.

WRONGLY CHOSEN LETTERS
See Spelling Mistakes — Ortographobia.

X (LETTER)
X-phobia (CP) — From the Greek letter X and the 24th letter of the English alphabet. The letter X is regarded as standing for "that which is unknown". In 1637, French philosopher René Descartes explained that X, Y and Z are to be used to represent what is unknown and are to correspond to A, B and C, used to represent what is known.[13]

X-RAYS
See Radiation (Medical Treatments) — Radiophobia.

YELLOW (COLOUR OR WORD)

Xanthophobia (NP) — From Greek *xantho* meaning "yellow or blonde".

YOUNG BOYS

See Boys — Boeiphobia.

YOUNG GIRLS

See Girls — Parthenophobia.

ZOMBIES

Zombiephobia (CP) — From West African *nzambi* meaning "god".

Chapter 20
Our Evolution in Phobia Understanding

"Why are we scared to die? Do any of us remember being scared when we were born?"

H.P. Lovecraft (1890–1937)

The word "phobia" has been used in psychiatry in the way we use it today only since the 19th century. Among the ancient writers who wrote of phobias while not using the term is the ancient Greek physician Hippocrates (c. 460–c. 370 BCE), "the father of medicine". He described a patient with what may be the first case of Sociophobia ever recorded. He writes of a man who "through bashfulness, suspicion and timorousness, will not be seen abroad ... he thinks every man observes him".[1]

IN ANCIENT TIMES

Before medicine was a well-organised curative discipline, people with illnesses went to philosophers for assistance. "It lay upon the philosophers to unwind the complications and to unearth the exact causes behind." Among the ancient philosophical interpretations of phobias was the Pythagorean interpretation. This held that phobias were "reminiscences" from former lives. An implication of this was that phobias had a religious association.[2]

"Phobia" was first used in the medical context by the early Roman medical writer Aulus Cornelius Celsus (c. 25 BCE–50 CE) to describe someone suffering from fear of water (Hydrophobia). The meaning of "phobia" has greatly expanded since then.

IN THE 16TH CENTURY

The famous 16th century French Renaissance essayist Michel de Montaigne (1533–1592) caustically observed in *Essais* (1580) that some "flee from the smell of apples more than from the dangers of gunfire. Others have become frightened by the sight of a mouse or cream." He further noted that "[a] man who fears suffering is already suffering from what he fears".

IN THE 17TH CENTURY

The fact that phobias may be learned was recognised in the 17th century by the famous French philosopher René Descartes (1596–1650). In 1650, Descartes wrote: "[F]rom whence proceed the passions which are peculiar to certain men ... the smell of roses may have caused some great headache in the child when it was in the cradle; or a cat may have affrighted it and none took notice of it, nor the child so much as remembered it; though the idea of that aversion he then had to roses or a cat remain imprinted in his brain to life live's end."[3]

Another Enlightenment personage who believed that phobias may be learned was the noted English philosopher John Locke (1632–1704). In 1671, Locke wrote: "A grown Person surfeiting with Honey, no sooner hears the Name of it, but his Phancy immediately carries Sickness and Qualms to his stomach, and he cannot bear the very *Idea* of it; other Ideas of Dislike and Sickness, and Vomiting presently accompany it, and he is disturb'd, but he knows from whence to date this Weakness, and can tell how he got this Indisposition: Had this happen'd to him, by an overdose of Honey, when a child, all the same Effects would have followed, but the Cause would have been mistaken, and the Antipathy counted Natural."[4]

IN THE 18TH CENTURY

In the 18th century, it was often believed that vertigo (dizziness) was "the dominant aspect" of phobias. French physician Francois Boissier de Sauvages de la Croix (1706–1767) called phobias *vertigo hysterique* and *vertigo hypocondriaque*. He reported the case of a woman who was afraid of falling and had attacks of vertigo — but only when she entered an empty church. A hundred years later the idea was still prominent. The dizziness was ascribed to a problem with the eye muscles.

One of the earliest attempts to comprehensively study phobias was by the French surgeon Antoine Le Camus (1722–1772). In his *Des Aversions* (1769), Le Camus classified the aversions (phobias) according to the five senses that might be affected — hearing, sight, smell, taste and touch. Le Camus also listed many clinical cases, including historical ones: Germanicus Caesar of ancient Rome and James I of England.

★ ★ ★

THE MOST POPULAR PHOBIA IN THE 18TH AND 19TH CENTURIES

If one were to estimate the "most popular" phobia in the 18th and 19th centuries, that distinction would probably go to Syphilophobia (fear of syphilis). By the 17th century it had already been described in the medical literature. What we today call Syphilophobia was then called "syphilitic mania" or *manie verolique*. The term "Syphilophobia" first appeared in a medical dictionary in 1848.

★ ★ ★

IN THE 19TH CENTURY

In the first half of the 19th century, phobias were only sporadically mentioned in medical textbooks and in the fledgling field of psychiatry. For example, a few phobias are listed by John Connolly (1794–1866) in his early psychiatry text, *An Inquiry Concerning the Indications of Insanity* (1830). In it, Connolly describes the case of a Russian general who was so afraid of mirrors that the Empress Catherine the Great "always took care to give him audience in a room without any".

The noted 19th century neurologist and psychiatrist Benedict Augustin Morel (1809–1873) described his own Acrophobia (fear of high places) in his *Traité des Dégénérescences Physiques, Intellectuelles et Morales de l'Espéce Humaine et des Causes qui Produisent ces Variétés Maladives* (1857). This may be the first occasion where a doctor describes his own phobia.

The first full clinical descriptions in their own right about what we would call phobic disorders today were presented by the pioneering German neurologist and psychiatrist Dr Carl Otto Freidrich Westphal (1800–1879). In 1871, Westphal described three male patients who feared going out into public places. The *agora* was the marketplace and assembly venue for public occasions in ancient Greece. Westphal coined the term "Agoraphobia" to refer to such a fear.[5]

The great Charles Darwin (1809–1882) addressed the issue of human fears in 1872. He suggested that fears have a function in natural selection and thus fear is a factor in human evolution. He observed that a fear that had survival value earlier in human history nevertheless may persist well past the time when it had such survival value.[6]

In 1876, French psychiatrist Legrand du Saulle (1830–1886) described a phobia as *peur des espaces* meaning "fear of spaces". He meant that a phobia created in the person's mind a boundary — one that could not be crossed. The person hesitates, trembles, breaks out into a sweat and cannot proceed.[7]

273

The pioneering English psychiatrist Henry Maudsley (1835–1918) in the third edition of his classic textbook, *The Pathology of Mind* (1879), wrote a fascinating account of an Agoraphobic patient. Maudsley classified all phobias as "melancholia". He also, astonishingly, advised against the naming of each phobia based upon its phobia source.[8]

Philosopher and psychologist William James (1842–1910) wrote of "pathological fears" and "certain peculiarities in the expression of ordinary fears". In his classic text, *The Principles of Psychology* (1890), he expressed the view that Agoraphobia may have had survival value in prehistoric humans but has no usefulness today.

Pioneering US psychologist G. Stanley Hall (1804–1884), "the father of child psychology", observed in 1897 that the "relative intensity (of different fear elements) fits past conditions better than it does present ones". This not only agreed with Darwin but also underscored the reality we have come to recognise as an essential part of a phobia — the intensity of the fear persists far beyond a reasonable expectation in time and space.[9]

By the end of the 19th century, there existed several detailed case histories of phobic disorders. In one of the best of these, in 1894, pioneering psychoanalyst Sigmund Freud (1856–1939) wrote a fascinating description of a patient with Agoraphobia. Freud stressed that phobias should be regarded primarily as symbols for other hidden fears. This was not always his view. Freud originally suggested an organic basis for phobias. He even believed that, as such, phobias were not amenable to psychotherapy. However, Freud later came to the view that at least some phobias had a psychological basis.

In 1895, Freud divided phobias into two groups according to the source of fear: 1) common phobias and 2) specific phobias. A common phobia was an exaggerated fear of all those things nearly everyone normally fears (death, night, snakes, illness, etc.). A specific phobia was a fear of special circumstances that inspire no fear in a normal person (public spaces, footpaths and sidewalks, the colour red, etc.). Freud then regarded phobias as part of an anxiety neurosis caused by "the accumulation of sexual tension produced by abstinence or by frustrated sexual excitation".[10]

IN THE 20TH CENTURY

In 1903, the French psychologist Pierre Janet (1859–1947) classified all neurotic disorders into two major divisions: Hysteria and Psychasthenia. Hysteria was any disturbance in sensation, movement and consciousness. Hysteria is still defined this way but since 1980 has been called "conversion disorder". Psychasthenia was any neurotic phenomenon, such as anxiety, compulsion, obsession, depression and phobia. "Psychasthenia" has dropped out of the psychologist's lexicon in more recent decades.

In 1913, the German psychiatrist Emil Kraepelin (1856–1926), who some argue is the father of modern psychiatry and who co-discovered Alzheimer's disease with Alois Alzheimer (1864–1915), presented the view that all phobias were the product of a diseased brain or a faulty metabolism. He fervently believed that eventually science would discover the organic cause of all mental disease.[11]

Doing the familiar or being in familiar surroundings reduces fear. We have known this for nearly a century. In a classic article by the founder of the behaviourist school of psychology, John Watson (1878–1958), the case of an 11-month-old boy called Albert was presented. Albert was "taught" to be phobic of harmless white rats. At first, Albert was not at all afraid of a white rat when it was placed before him. Then, whenever a white rat was placed before him, Watson rang a bell with a deafening sound that frightened Albert. Eventually, Albert began to cry as soon as he merely saw a white rat. In addition, Albert had a strong tendency to place his thumb in his mouth as soon as he was frightened. Watson was able to condition Albert so that he did not become afraid as long as his thumb remained in his mouth. Another classic study in psychology described the case of a child who showed no fear of strange objects as long as she was sitting in her own familiar high chair. However, the same fear stimuli caused fear reactions when she was sitting on the floor. Interestingly, other psychologists have argued that Watson may have overstated his claims. Attempts at repeating his "Albert" experiments with other children have not always produced the same results. Still, we humans do need our security blankets, don't we?[12]

Psychoanalysts of the mid-20th century assumed that all phobias hid from the patient the real, unconscious source of the underlying anxiety. It was believed by some that this resembled dream symbolism, so much a characteristic of psychoanalysis, in which the content of a dream is construed to be a facade behind which are concealed the latent thoughts that truly call for the anxiety.[13]

★ ★ ★

"THE OPEN DOOR" TO PHOBIAS
The year 1966 was an important year in the history of phobias. In that year the world's first phobia organisation was formed. It was called "The Open Door" but later changed its name to PAX — the Latin term for "peace" — in this case, peace of mind.

★ ★ ★

In the first six decades of the 20th century, phobias were sometimes explained as being caused by hereditary factors, poor upbringing, stomach ailments, and general brain or body functioning problems. Most medical authorities still failed to separate the phobic disorders from other conditions that gave rise to delusion fears.

At the end of the 1960s, many experts in the field believed that only about one in 10 people suffered from a phobia. For example, three researchers led by Dr Stewart Agras of Stanford University reported in 1969 that about 77 out of 1,000 people suffer from some type of phobic disorder. They added that fears of illness or injury are the most common phobias, while Agoraphobia is the most frequent phobia for which individuals seek treatment.[14]

In the 1970s, there was a prominent view that new fears may be acquired by a simple classical conditioning process in which a neutral stimulus is paired with, or shortly before, a noxious stimulus — this is learning by temporal contiguity. The new fear increases with the frequency of the pairing, with the strength of the noxious stimulus, and when the pairing occurs in conditions of confinement or when nothing can be done to stop the noxious stimulation. Once acquired, fear may be used as a drive to motivate instrumental learning since a sudden reduction in the strength of fear serves as a reward to reinforce such learning — this is learning by drive reduction. People can acquire fears rapidly by modelling or by simply being told that a given situation is frightening, without their ever experiencing any noxious stimulus themselves — this is vicarious learning. By this logic, anything may be the object of a phobic stimulus. That is why the list of phobias is so long.

★ ★ ★

PHOBIC DISORDERS AND PHOBIC NEUROSES
Phobic disorders used to be called phobic neuroses. But the "neuroses" label was dropped from the DSM-III-R in the mid-1980s.[15]

★ ★ ★

PHOBICS AND PHOBIC WORDS
Brain studies have found that compared with non-phobics, phobics are more hypersensitive even to the mentioning of phobia names. This is the finding of German clinicians at the Friedrich-Schiller University in Jena, led by Dr T. Straube.[16]

* * *

Phobic reactions can be learned from the positive or negative consequences that are experienced. US psychologist Orval Hobart Mowrer (1907–1982) theorised that two factors were involved in "operant conditioning". First, the phobia develops through exposure to the stimulus. Second, it is maintained by avoidance behaviour (operant) of the stimulus. There is no opportunity to reduce the anxiety through experience. This results in a "self-defeating" situation Mowrer termed "neurotic paradox".[17]

"THE DISGUST FACTOR" IN PHOBIAS

It has been observed by clinicians that some phobias seem to be more difficult to understand and treat compared with others. One psychologist believes that separate emotions of revulsion towards the phobic stimulus — "the disgust factor" — may explain this. Dr Jeffrey Lohr notes that, for instance, there is often a strong "yuck" response to blood, vomit and needles associated with surgery. "Researchers who treat phobia as a matter of simple fear may do so to their client's peril. If you're looking to try to change the behaviour, there may be different mechanisms for changing loathing than for changing fear." Dr Lohr and colleagues conducted a series of experiments attempting to separate "the disgust factor" in the phobias of various patients. They created images that might elicit fear, disgust, or fear and disgust together, including images of rotting food, faeces and surgeries, along with images that depicted neutral scenes, such as piles of tools or kitchen utensils. The subjects were then shown an image on the left side of a screen for about eight seconds and a facial expression on the right side of the screen for about two seconds. The facial expressions showed images of people expressing disgust (nose wrinkled, mouth scrunched up, eyes squeezed shut), fear (eyes and mouth open wide) or neutrality. Each picture was paired at different times with each facial expression.

When asked to rate what per cent of the time each face was paired with a picture, subjects paired the "disgusting" images with both fearful and disgusted expressions, and the rotting foods and bodily function images with disgusted expressions. The subjects also paired the neutral expressions with neutral images. They did this even though each image was shown with each expression the same number of times. According to Dr Lohr, "Their perceptions were inaccurate. They were associating the expressions in a biased manner with what they perceived to be the disgusting or fearful object."[18]

PHOBIAS AND HEART DISEASE IN WOMEN

According to a Harvard University study, women with phobias such as the fear of enclosed spaces, heights or open spaces are at a higher risk of suffering fatal heart attacks than women with fewer or no phobias. Dr Christine Albert says that previous studies have shown that phobias in men are associated with greater heart-disease risk. The same seems to be true for women. In the study using a survey following women over many years, women who expressed a higher level of phobia anxiety when first surveyed had a 59 per cent increased risk of suffering a sudden cardiac death.[19]

THE MOLECULAR MECHANISM OF FEAR FOUND?

MIT researchers believe they have uncovered the molecular mechanism that governs the formation of fears stemming from traumatic events. This research could lead to the first drug to treat the millions of adults who suffer each year from persistent and debilitating fears and phobias. Kinases are enzymes that change proteins and are an important part of the biochemistry of the brain. Dr Li-Huei Tsai and colleagues have demonstrated in their experiments with mice that inhibiting a kinase called Cdk5 helps the extinction of fear learned in a particular context.

On the other hand, the learned fear persisted when the activity of this kinase was increased in the hippocampus. The hippocampus is the centre of the brain, which is theorised as the major brain region for storing memories. According to Dr Tsai, "Remarkably, inhibiting Cdk5 facilitated extinction of learned fear in mice. These data point to a promising therapeutic avenue to treat emotional disorders and raises hope for patients suffering from post-traumatic stress disorder or phobia."[20]

CAN A PHOBIA OR FEAR REALLY MAKE YOUR BLOOD FREEZE IN YOUR VEINS?

There may be some truth in the expressions "The blood froze in my veins" and "My blood curdled". German researchers have discovered that phobias, intense fears and panic attacks can not only really make our blood clot but can increase the risk of heart attack and stroke. For several years we have known that anxiety and stress can influence blood coagulation. Drs Franziska Geiser and Ursula Harbrecht conducted a very careful examination of coagulation in patients with phobias and other intense fears, and compared them to a control group without such phobias and intense fears. All subjects had blood drawn. They were then directed to perform tasks on a computer. Some computer images induced fear in subjects. The researchers found that "[t]he group of anxiety patients showed a much more highly activated coagulation system than the healthy control group". A highly activated coagulation system of this kind is not healthy. In extreme cases this can lead to the blockage of a coronary artery. Drs Geiser and Harbrecht contend that "this increased coagulation tendency could be the 'missing link' that explains why anxiety patients have a statistically higher risk of dying from heart disease by a factor of three or four. Of course, this doesn't mean that every patient with a marked anxiety disorder must now worry about having a heart attack. The coagulation values we measured were always within the physiological scale, which means there is no acute danger."[21]

COULD PHOBIAS BE EMBEDDED IN OUR DNA?

Scientists in the field of evolutionary biology believe that phobias may very well be embedded in our DNA. This view was put forward by Drs A. Ohman and S. Mineka from the Karolinska Institutet in Stockholm, Sweden, in 2001. They pointed out that fears of snakes, spiders, sharks and other animals that could hurt us correspond to that which poses a threat to our evolutionary survival, are the most easily triggered and are often the hardest fears to unlearn. They add that it may or may not be coincidental that all of the animals that earn widespread panic evolved before humans. Although many of the big mammals we often fear reached their recognisable current forms during or after the Pleistocene epoch (2.5 million to 12,000 years ago), thus allowing humans to be more adapted to them, spiders, snakes and sharks all developed before the Cretacian period (145 to 65 million years ago). This was just as primates were beginning to evolve. So, perhaps the fear of such animals as spiders, snakes and sharks is embedded in our earliest neurons and DNA. On the other hand, they note that phobias vary from culture to culture and have been shown to respond to cultural factors. For example, the fear of sharks was at an all-time high after the release of *Jaws* in 1975.[22]

Chapter 21
Treatment

"He had one peculiar weakness; he had faced death in many forms but he had never faced a dentist."

H.G. Wells (1866–1947), *Bealby*

It is natural to have a little fear. According to Dr Jerilyn Ross, director of the Ross Center for Anxiety and Related Disorders in Washington, DC, "Some level of anxiety helps warn us when there is danger or motivates us to behave in a certain way. It is healthy." More often than not, people with phobias know their reactions are not rational. They are well aware that the plane probably will not crash, the dog will not bite or the lift will not get stuck. But Dr Ross says that "throwing statistics at them will not help. They say, 'I don't understand why, but I feel like if I do it, I'll die.'"[1]

The treatment of choice among most therapists today focuses on helping people cope with phobic reactions in their lives. In doing this, therapists use an integrated approach involving a combination of several forms of therapy: behaviour therapy, exposure therapy, flooding, group therapy, hypnotherapy, eye movement desensitisation and reprocessing (EMDR), and medications.

Behaviour therapy
Behaviour therapy today is based upon the premise that a phobia is a learned response. As such, it can be unlearned as well. The work of South African psychologist John Wolpe (1915–1997) on reciprocal

inhibition laid the foundation for the current view that through a number of behavioural therapeutic techniques, the phobic response can be reduced or eliminated.

Exposure therapy
Exposure therapy may be mild or intense. The patient is exposed to the phobic stimulus either by means of a photo or by means of the stimulus itself at a distance.

Flooding
A more intense form of exposure therapy is called "flooding". Essentially, this is the equivalent of throwing the person into the deep end of the pool rather than having them wade in slowly from the shallow end.

Group therapy
Group therapy is a form of psychotherapy in which the therapist, rather than treating one individual, treats a group of individuals with the same or similar condition.

Hypnotherapy
Hypnotherapy involves the patient being placed under hypnosis, during which time hypnotic suggestions may be put to them. "Hypnosis" is from the Greek *hynos* meaning "sleep".

Eye movement desensitisation and reprocessing (EMDR)
EMDR involves imagined exposure to the phobic source along with specific eye movements that attempt to stimulate the brain to better process the phobic stimulus. This approach was developed by US psychologist Francine Shapiro (1954–) to resolve the development of trauma-related disorders resulting from combat, rape or other such distressing events.

Medications

A number of medications, chiefly antidepressants and benzodiazepines, are sometimes involved in the treatment of phobias. However, they are not used on their own.

There is little doubt that phobias do occasionally disappear by themselves or after recall of a forgotten trauma that had initiated the phobia.[2]

* * *

A 2007 review of studies of treatments for specific phobias found that "[a] few studies suggest that virtual reality may be effective in flying and height phobia, but this needs to be substantiated by more controlled trials. Cognitive therapy is most helpful in Claustrophobia, and Blood-injury phobia is uniquely responsive to applied tension. The limited data on medication have not been promising with the exception of adjunctive D-clycoserine." The authors of the review, led by Dr Y. Choy from the New York State Psychiatric Institute in New York City, stress that much more research is needed in order to establish the best treatments for different phobias.[3]

* * *

Fears are more easily extinguished when the phobic stimulus is "massed" rather than when it is received over a longer period of time. "Massing" occurs when the phobic stimulus is experienced numerous times over a short period of time. In experiments with mice conducted at UCLA, under the direction of Dr Mark Barad, scientists discovered that when, let us say, 10 exposures to the phobic stimulus occur over one hour compared with 10 exposures over 10 hours, the fear is easier to treat and thus overcome in the first instance rather than the second. It is an illustration of the mice "putting their fears behind them", so to speak. If it is true for mice, it may be true for people too.[4]

YOHIMBINE TO TREAT PHOBIAS?

Some researchers believe they have demonstrated that yohimbine, a substance found in yohimbe tree bark, acts to accelerate recovery from anxiety disorders. In the latest in a series of studies of how mice acquire, express and extinguish conditioned fear, UCLA scientists found that yohimbine helps mice learn to overcome the fear faster by enhancing the effects of the natural release of adrenaline. Adrenaline prompts physiological changes, such as increased heart and metabolism rates, in response to physical and mental stress. In a study led by Dr Mark Barad, mice treated with yohimbine overcame their fears four times as fast as those treated with propanolol. Propanolol is a medication commonly used to treat symptoms of anxiety disorders by blunting the physiological effects of adrenaline.[5]

FEW PEOPLE GET TREATMENT FOR PHOBIAS

According to Professor Gavin Andrews, head of clinical research for anxiety and depression at St Vincent's Hospital in Sydney, one in 12 Australians suffer from a phobia but few people get treatment. In a recent review of phobia research, Professor Andrews showed that only 24 per cent of Australians with Agoraphobia and only 7 per cent of Australians with Sociophobia received effective treatment, with the figure for other phobias lower still.[6]

* * *

SELF-HELP TREATMENTS BENEFICIAL
Australian researchers suggest that certain self-help treatments for social anxiety disorder (Sociophobia) may be just as effective as more traditional "therapist only" treatments. According to Dr Ron Rapee, professor of psychology at Macquarie University in Sydney,

data from the Australian Bureau of Statistics (1997 National Survey of Health and Wellbeing) states that Sociophobia affects more than 200,000 Australians every year. Of these people, 80 per cent do not seek treatment. However, the results of a Macquarie University self-help treatment trial for Sociophobia yielded "promising news for both anxiety sufferers and mental health services". The Macquarie study, led by Dr Rapee, investigated the efficacy of pure self-help through written materials for severe Sociophobia and self-help augmented by five group sessions with a therapist. These conditions were compared with a waiting-list control and standard, therapist-led group therapy. Dr Rapee adds, "Such methods may provide a template for a highly resource-effective method of treatment delivery. Mental health services around the world are limited in their reach and scope. In addition, a large proportion of people with anxiety disorders including Sociophobia do not seek help from traditional mental health services, rather they prefer to deal with difficulties themselves. For these people in particular, self-help might provide an acceptable alternative to traditional therapy."[7]

* * *

THE HOLY GRAIL OF PHOBIA TREATMENT FOUND?

It has been called the Holy Grail of phobia treatment. Researchers have developed a non-invasive technique to block the return of fear memories in humans. The technique may change how we view the storage processes of memory and could lead to new ways to treat phobias and other anxiety disorders. Science has long sought to understand fear memories. These are expressed as the emotional reaction of the body to objects or events previously linked to potential danger. It is known that such emotional responses could dissipate over time (extinction) in which the same event is experienced in a safe environment. After extinction, the fear memory is merely suppressed, not erased, and therefore these memories could resurface under certain conditions, such as unrelated stress. This is the foundation of post-traumatic stress disorder. In some cases, the re-emergence of the emotional memory is maladaptive, leading to anxiety disorders. Mindful of this, researchers have sought ways to prevent the return of fear memories. While researchers have traditionally seen long-term memory as fixed and resistant, it is now becoming clear that memory is, in fact, dynamic and flexible. As a result, the act of remembering makes the memory vulnerable until it is stored again. This is a process called "reconsolidation". During reconsolidation, new information can be incorporated into the old memory. This was the phase during which a team of New York University researchers, led by psychologist Dr Elizabeth Phelps, sought to employ a technique to block the return of fear memories. The Phelps team showed that reactivating fear memories in humans allows them to be updated with non-fearful information. As a result, fear responses no longer return.

In order to achieve this, the researchers created a fear memory by showing participants a visual object and pairing it with mild electric shocks. Once this fear memory was formed, participants were reminded of the object a day later. This reactivation of the memory was intended to initiate the reconsolidation process. During this process, information that the same object was now "safe" was provided through extinction training. Presenting this new "safe" information during reconsolidation was designed to incorporate it into the initial fear memory. A day later, the participants were tested again to see whether they continued to demonstrate a fear response when presented with the object. It was discovered that extinction training on its own led to the reduction of fear, but fear returned when tested at a later time or after the participant was under stress. However, the Phelps team found that if extinction training was conducted during the reconsolidation window, when the memory was temporarily unstable, fear responses did not return. They also showed that rewriting of the fear memory as safe was specific to the object that was reactivated prior to extinction. Fear memories for other objects returned following extinction, suggesting that the technique is selective rather than having a general effect on memories. In all, the experiment was conducted over three days. The memory was formed in the first day, rewritten on the second day, and tested for fear on the third day. However, to examine how enduring this effect is, some participants were tested again about a year later. Even after this period of time, the fear memory did not return in those subjects who had extinction during the reconsolidation window. These results suggest that the old fear memory was changed from its original form and that this change persists over time.[8]

CAN A PAINKILLER KILL A PHOBIA TOO?

It may be possible one day to cure your phobia through an injection. This is the prediction of two Japanese researchers, Drs Masayuki Yoshida and Ruriko Hirano from the University of Hiroshima, who have studied the cerebellum. This is an area of the brain that they believe is involved with the development and storage of our fears. Using classical conditioning techniques, fish were taught to become afraid of a light flashed in their eyes. By administering a low-voltage electric shock every time a light was shone, the fish were taught to associate the light with being shocked. Dr Yoshida explains: "As you would expect, the goldfish we used in our study soon became afraid of the flash of light because, whether or not we actually gave them a shock, they had quickly learned to expect one. Fear was demonstrated by their heartbeats decreasing, in a similar way to how our heart rate increases when someone gives us a fright." Dr Yoshida contends that humans can also be "trained" to become afraid. In fact, simple classical conditioning is rooted in our childhood and early development and can explain many of our behaviours. However, in this study, the researchers also discovered that fish that had first been injected in the cerebellum with lidocaine (a painkiller) had stable heart rates and showed no fear when the light was shone. They were prevented from learning to become afraid. While humans are not goldfish, Drs Yoshida and Hirano hope that with further study it may soon be possible to understand more about the biological and chemical processes that cause us to become afraid.[9]

Chapter 22
Childhood Phobias

"Fear of disease killed more men than disease itself."
Mohandas K. Gandhi (1869–1948)

It is probably safe to say that every child has fears in varying degrees. Some are the normal fears of childhood while others are not. It is the role of the parent or teacher to reassure a frightened youngster. The ability to do this well can result in the child feeling secure and safe in their present and later life.

A certain amount of fear is healthy and understandable. It keeps us and our children out of harm's way. We teach our children to fear running into a busy street, accepting candy from strangers, swallowing unidentified substances from the medicine cabinet, etc. In such cases, we are teaching our children to fear the results. We are, in essence, teaching them caution, which is quite a different matter from dealing with a youngster who is responding to an imaginary rather than a real danger. Such a child evidencing anxiety when there doesn't seem to be anything specific to be anxious about, whose fear is so great, borders on becoming phobic.

As with adulthood (see Chapter 1), the list of the most common phobias in childhood is difficult to determine. Based upon years of reports by both children and parents, the 30 most common phobias in childhood look something like this (in alphabetical order):

1) Alone (Being Alone) (Eremophobia)

2) Angry People (Cholerophobia)

3) Blood (Haematophobia)

4) Corpses (Necrophobia)

5) Darkness (Achluophobia)

6) Death (Thanatophobia)

7) Death of a Parent (Thanatophobia)

8) Deformed People (Dysmorphophobia)

9) Dentists (Dentophobia)

10) Dogs (Caninophobia)

11) Drowning (Aquaphobia)

12) Embarrassment (Sociophobia)

13) Failure (Atychiphobia)

14) Flying (Flying in an Aircraft) (Aviophobia)

15) High Places (Acrophobia)

16) Injections (Trypanophobia)

17) Lightning (Keraunophobia)

18) Mistakes (Hamartophobia)

19) Pain (One's Own) (Algophobia)

20) Pointed Objects (Aichmophobia)

21) Police (Policiphobia)

22) Public Speaking (Glossophobia)

23) Rejection (Including by Peers) (Rejectuphobia)

24) Reptiles (Herpetophobia)

25) Ridicule (Catagelophobia)

26) Snakes (Ophidiophobia)

27) Spiders (Arachnophobia)

28) Tests (Academic) (Examinaphobia)

29) Thunder (Brontophobia)

30) Vomiting (Emetophobia)

Many of these fears, if not recognised and treated properly in children, can develop into more serious phobias in adult life.

HOW EARLY CAN A PHOBIA DEVELOP?

It is unknown how early a phobia can develop. A phobia may develop before a person is aware of it and certainly long before they can describe it with words. We have observed human infants as young as five days of age recognise the edge of a board if they are placed on it. At six months of age they take action to avoid the edge. If they can, they will crawl away from the edge of a board on which they are placed. We assume that the motivation is to seek safety. If they attempt to move to safety, that in itself is evidence of some anxiety and the presence of fear.[1]

RACHMAN'S THREE PATHWAYS THEORY

In 1961, Canadian psychologist Stanley Rachman (1934–) argued that children acquire phobias by one of three pathways: direct conditioning, modelling or instructions/information. Australian researchers have presented evidence that Rachman's theory is probably right with respect to children's Caninophobia and probably right with respect to other children's phobias.[2]

CAN WE TRANSMIT PHOBIAS TO OUR CHILDREN?

For nearly five decades there has been solid scientific evidence that humans can transmit phobias through modelling. "Modelling" essentially means "by example". It has been shown that the degree of the modelling effect producing a fear reaction is proportional to the degree of stress during the observed situation. The more frightened person A is when person B sees them, the more intense is the modelling effect in person B and the more likely that person B will also become fearful of what frightened person A. If person B also experiences stress as they see person A experience fear, this increases person B's fear even more.[3]

292

* * *

IS FOOD NEOPHOBIA INHERITED?
Food Neophobia (fear of new foods) in children has long been associated with low consumption of healthy foods, such as protein foods, fruits and vegetables. Many child development authorities, not to mention many parents, had always assumed that the resultant food rejection by children is a normal part of childhood. Parents were advised to model desirable eating habits so children would get the message. The theory behind this is that parental good eating behaviour will create a good eating example — that environment determines food Neophobia. New light was shed on this issue by a team of University of London researchers. They claim to have discovered evidence that food Neophobia in children is genetic in nature and not environmental. Interesting idea for why little Michael hates broccoli.[4]

* * *

CAN WE ELIMINATE PHOBIAS IN CHILDREN?

Not long after John Watson presented the case of little Albert and demonstrated how a phobia could be produced in a child, another psychologist, Mary Cover Jones, demonstrated how a phobia could be eliminated in a child. Peter was a three-year-old boy whose fear of white rats extended to white rabbits, white fur coats, white feathers and cotton wool. By associating the white rabbit with food the child enjoyed and placing the child among other children who did not have a fear of white rabbits, she was able to recondition the child out of the phobia using the reverse of Watson's conditioning techniques. The seven steps of eliminating phobias in children that were formulated by Jones constitute the foundation of modern techniques used to eliminate phobias.[5]

* * *

CHILDREN CURED OF PHOBIA IN ONE-SESSION TREATMENT
Fifty-five per cent of children who underwent an intensive one-session treatment of three hours were freed from their phobia. The treatment is quick and cost-effective with no side effects. The treatment form is also culture-neutral so does not need to be adapted to the country or the place in which it is to be used. Psychologist Dr Lena Reuterskiold of Stockholm, Sweden, who utilises this form of treatment, says, "Children who are not cured of their phobias run a great risk of developing other areas of anxiety later on. It's therefore important to find effective forms of treatment that can reduce this risk. The method we have now tested also functions for other types of phobias. In a one-session treatment the children, together with their therapist, gradually approach what they are afraid of in a controlled and planned manner. The therapist describes and carefully demonstrates before the child is allowed to try. Because the children remain in the anxiety-inducing situation, they can experience how their anxiety and fear abates and how the expected catastrophe in fact does not occur. With the patient remaining in the situation for an extended period, without running away, new learning occurs, producing a development toward a new behaviour. This is all done on a voluntary basis, which is also a precondition for successful treatment." Dr Reuterskiold contends that "[o]ne-session treatment has also proven to be effective over time. Adults who have been treated with this method have been able to notice the effects of the treatment more than a year after the session. And nothing indicates that the effect would taper off sooner in children, which we assume will soon be confirmed by a follow-up study."[6]

* * *

DO MEDICATIONS WORK IN TREATING CHILDHOOD PHOBIAS?

Medications for treating mental health conditions are steadily improving. One of the first major studies to indicate that medications may work in treating children and adolescents suffering from phobias was a 2001 study conducted by the US National Institute of Mental Health (NIMH). It found that one particular medication (Fluvoxamine) was more than twice as effective as a placebo in helping children and adolescents overcome anxiety disorders, including phobias. The study involved 128 children and adolescents aged between six and 17 years over a period of eight weeks. Symptoms improved in 76 per cent of those randomly assigned to take the medication, compared with only 29 per cent of those in the placebo group. The study pointed out that anxiety disorders affect an estimated 13 per cent of children and adolescents during any given six-month period. As such, this makes them the most common class of psychiatric disorders in that age group, yet the disorders are often not recognised and most who have them do not receive treatment. The study found that anxiety disorders, including phobias, "are properly recognised through a careful evaluation that includes direct examination of the child, a parent interview and a collection of past history" as they "cause significant suffering and functional impairment in the affected children". The study adds that "[w]hile not all of them will continue to suffer from these disorders into adulthood, some will, and early treatment may help prevent future mental health problems ..."[7]

SCHOOL-PHOBIA

School-phobia has received much community attention and been studied quite often in recent years. Among the many things we know about the topic, it has been found that, compared with children who are merely anxious about school, children who are genuinely School-phobic "had a later age of onset and showed more pervasive (severe) school refusal than separation-anxious school refusers".[8]

SPIDER FEARS

Children are commonly very afraid of spiders (Arachnophobia). A 1996 Netherlands study of 22 children with Arachnophobia found that "[w]hile 46 per cent of the children claimed to have always been afraid, 41 per cent ascribed the onset of their fear to aversion conditioning events. The large majority of these events were confirmed by parents. These findings cast doubts on a strong version of the non-associative account of spider phobia, i.e., the idea that spider phobia is acquired in the complete absence of learning experiences." A 1997 study by the same team of researchers found that "[c]hildren who reported 'none', 'some' or 'a lot' of spider fear were compared with each other in terms of pathways [the course to their behaviour]. No differences between the three groups were found with respect to the frequency of modelling and information experiences. However, highly fearful children more often reported conditioning experiences than low or moderate fearful children."[9]

SOME STRATEGIES TO DEAL WITH COMMON CHILDHOOD PHOBIAS

Fear of Darkness (Achluophobia) in Childhood
Generally, fear of the dark occurs when parents insist that the child stay in a totally darkened room at bedtime or when the child wakes up in the middle of the night. Some children are so terrified by the dark that their heartbeats actually increase. Parents need to recognise the fact that the room looks totally different to the child when the lights are out, and should take steps to reassure the youngster, even if the fear seems completely irrational to them.

1) Use a night light but experiment with its placement to be sure that it does not create all sorts of frightening shadows.

2) After the light has been turned out, stay in the room for a few minutes and talk about how different things look. A curtain blowing in the breeze looks very different at night than it does during the daytime.

3) Leave the door to the child's room slightly open and tell them that you will not be far away.

4) When the child is in middle childhood and awakens during the night, do not invite them into your bed or you risk starting a habit that is difficult to break. Instead, comfort them in their own room and tell them that you are proud of them for being grown up enough to sleep in a room by themselves.

5) Remain consistent in your approach to their behaviour.

Fear of Dogs (Caninophobia), Reptiles (Herpetophobia) and Snakes (Ophidiophobia) in Childhood
While the fear of animals affects almost all children, it happily seems to decrease as the child gets older. In the intervening years, a number of approaches can lessen the child's fears.

1) Don't transmit your own fear. Study and then teach the youngster the proper behaviour around animals. For example, always approach a dog from the front, where it can see and sniff your hand.

2) Identify the child's fear for them. For example, "Dogs can be scary, but this one lives right next door, and he wants to be your friend."

3) Have the child mingle with other children and their pets so they can see others feeling comfortable around animals.

4) Under no circumstances should any child (or adult, for that matter) be allowed to tease or mistreat an animal. This can provoke an attack

or a bite. If a child sees this, then it will doubtless be a considerable time before the youngster's fears can be fully overcome.

5) Don't force the child to pet an animal. Let them do it in their own good time. Don't encourage hand-feeding animals whose bite may be bigger than the portion offered.

Fear of the Dentist (Dentophobia) in Childhood

Clearly this is often an unresolved fear from childhood since so many adults are fearful of going to the dentist. It is usually provoked because the child feels they have absolutely no control over the situation. It's a fact of life that children do need to go to the dentist at regular intervals so their fear must be dealt with and overcome.

1) Do some research to find a dentist who has a good manner with children.
2) Start early so the child will get used to visiting the dentist's office for simple checkups when nothing except a cursory examination is required.
3) Teach the child good dental hygiene so that trips to the dentist will be minimal.
4) Try not to transmit your own fears of the dentist to children.

Fear of Death (Thanatophobia) in Childhood

Children are usually curious about death and this is normal unless the child begins to suddenly worry that someone they love will die soon. The average child generally doesn't really fear death until they have experienced the death of a person or animal. It is then that they may feel the first inklings of their mortality.

1) Be willing to discuss death with children if they wish it, but use this as a time for reassurance, indicating that they really need not worry about it right now.

2) Be honest when someone close to the child dies through illness or accident. It's the child's lack of knowledge that will cause their fears.

3) Be reassuring if the child thinks they were responsible for a death. This can sometimes happen. Youngsters when angry can think, "I hate him. I wish he were dead." If by some awful chance the person to whom the hate was directed dies, the child can feel responsible. Be sure that the child knows they are not to blame.

4) Many experts feel that a child should be over five years of age before they are exposed to a funeral home or funeral service and only then if they are willing. You should describe what is happening as being a way of saying goodbye.

Chapter 23
Phobias of the Famous

"Men fear death as children fear to go in the dark."
Sir Francis Bacon (1561–1626)

The following is a list of phobias allegedly suffered by the famous. Some people are historical figures while others are modern celebrities.

Agassi, Andre (29 April 1970–)
Spiders (Arachnophobia)

Alexander the Great (356–323 BCE)
Cats (Felinophobia)

Ali, Muhammad (17 January 1942–)
Flying (Flying in an Aircraft) (Aviophobia)

Allen, Lily (2 May 1985–)
Stage (The Stage) (Topophobia)

Allen, Woody (1 December 1935–)
Bad People (Scelerophobia)
Cancer (Carcinomatophobia)
Children (Paedophobia)
Colours (Chromophobia)
Crowds (Ochlophobia)
Daylight (Phengophobia)
Deer (Alkephobia)
Disease (Nosophobia)

Dogs (Caninophobia)
Elevators (Elevatuphobia)
Enclosed Spaces (Claustrophobia)
High Places (Acrophobia)
Insects (Entomophobia)
Pleasure (Hedonophobia)
Poison (Toxicophobia)
Public Places (Agoraphobia)
Social Situations (Sociophobia)
Tunnels (Tubuphobia)
Uncleanliness (Rhypophobia)

Anderson, Pamela (1 July 1967–)
Mirrors (Eisoptrophobia)

Aniston, Jennifer (11 February 1969–)
Flying (Flying in an Aircraft) (Aviophobia)

Armstrong, Neil (30 August 1930–)
Social Situations (Sociophobia)

Asimov, Isaac (2 January 1920–6 April 1992)
Flying (Flying in an Aircraft) (Aviophobia)

Baez, Joan (9 January 1941–)
Vomiting (Emetophobia)

Ball, Lucille (6 August 1911–26 April 1989)
Social Situations (Sociophobia)

Banks, Tyra (4 December 1973–)
Marine Mammals (Cetusaphobia)

Bardot, Brigitte (28 September 1934–)
Alone (Being Alone) (Eremophobia)

Barker, Travis (14 November 1975–)
Flying (Flying in an Aircraft) (Aviophobia)

Barrymore, Drew (22 February 1975–)
Enclosed Spaces (Claustrophobia)

Barton, Clara (25 December 1821–12 April 1912)
Social Situations (Sociophobia)

Basinger, Kim (8 December 1953–)
Public Places (Agoraphobia)
Public Speaking (Glossophobia)

Bean, Sean (17 April 1959–)
Flying (Flying in an Aircraft) (Aviophobia)

Beckham, David (2 May 1975–)
Birds (Ornithophobia)
Disorder (Ataxiophobia)

Behr, Dani (9 July 1970–)
Jumping (Catapedaphobia)

Benjamin, Lucy (25 June 1970–)
Insects (Entomophobia)

Bergkamp, Dennis (10 May 1969–)
Flying (Flying in an Aircraft) (Aviophobia)

Bergman, Ingrid (29 August 1915–29 August 1982)
Social Situations (Sociophobia)

Biel, Jessica (3 March 1982–)
Aging (Aetatemophobia)

Bloom, Orlando (13 January 1977–)
Pigs (Porcuphobia)

Bonaparte, Napoleon (15 August 1769–5 May 1821)
Cats (Felinophobia)

Boreanaz, David (16 May 1969–)
Enclosed Spaces (Claustrophobia)
Fish (Icthyophobia)
High Places (Acrophobia)
Waterfalls (Casicarephobia)

Bowie, David (8 January 1947–)
Social Situations (Sociophobia)

Bradbury, Ray (22 August 1920–)
Flying (Flying in an Aircraft) (Aviophobia)

Brockovich, Erin (22 June 1960–)
Social Situations (Sociophobia)

Brooker, Charlie (3 March 1971–)
Vomiting (Emetophobia)

Bugner, Joe (13 March 1950–)
Flying (Flying in an Aircraft) (Aviophobia)

Bunyan, John (28 November 1628–31 August 1688)
Churches (Ecclesiophobia)

Burnley, Benjamin (10 March 1978–)
Flying (Flying in an Aircraft) (Aviophobia)

Caesar, Augustus (23 September 63 BCE–19 August 14 CE)
Cats (Felinophobia)
Darkness (Achulophobia)
Lightning (Keraunophobia)

Caesar, Germanicus (24 May 16 or 15 BCE–10 October 19 CE)
Chickens (Alektorophobia)

Caesar, Julius (13 July 100–15 March 44 BCE)
Cats (Felinophobia)

Cain, Dean (31 July 1966–)
Flying (Flying in an Aircraft) (Aviophobia)

Carpenter, Mary Chapin (21 February 1958–)
Social Situations (Sociophobia)

Carrey, Jim (17 January 1962–)
Social Situations (Sociophobia)

Carson, Johnny (23 October 1925–23 January 2005)
Social Situations (Sociophobia)

Carver, Raymond (25 May 1938–2 August 1988)
Social Situations (Sociophobia)

Cash, Johnny (26 February 1932–12 September 2003)
Flying (Flying in an Aircraft) (Aviophobia)
Snakes (Ophidiophobia)

Chase, Chevy (8 October 1943–)
Snakes (Ophidiophobia)

Chasez, J.C. (8 August 1976–)
Injections (Trypanophobia)

Cheever, John (27 May 1912–18 June 1982)
Bridges (Gephyrophobia)

Cher (20 May 1946–)
Flying (Flying in an Aircraft) (Aviophobia)
Social Situations (Sociophobia)

Christie, Agatha (15 September 1890–12 January 1976)
Public Speaking (Glossophobia)
Social Situations (Sociophobia)

Cole, Cheryl (30 June 1983–)
Cotton (Xylinalinaphobia)

Combs, Sean "Diddy" (4 November 1969–)
Clowns (Coulrophobia)

Connery, Sean (25 August 1930–)
Red (Colour or Word) (Ereuthrophobia)

Costner, Kevin (18 January 1955–)
Social Situations (Sociophobia)

Cox, Courtney (16 June 1964–)
Social Situations (Sociophobia)

Crawford, Joan (23 March 1905–10 May 1977)
Germs (Spermophobia)

Crow, Sheryl (11 February 1962–)
High Places (Acrophobia)
Noises (Ligyrophobia)

Cruise, Tom (3 July 1962–)
Bald (Being or Becoming Bald) (Phalacrophobia)
Social Situations (Sociophobia)

Culkin, Macaulay (26 August 1980–)
Public Places (Agoraphobia)

Curtis, Tony (3 June 1925–29 September 2010)
Flying (Flying in an Aircraft) (Aviophobia)

D'Acampo, Gino (17 July 1975–)
Insects (Entomophobia)

Dallerup, Camilla (6 April 1974–)
Insects (Entomophobia)
Spiders (Arachnophobia)

De Niro, Robert (17 August 1943–)
Dentists (Dentophobia)
Social Situations (Sociophobia)

Deen, Paula (19 January 1947–)
Public Places (Agoraphobia)

Demosthenes (384–322 BCE)
Stage (The Stage) (Topophobia)

Depp, Johnny (9 June 1963–)
Clowns (Coulrophobia)
Spectres (Spectrophobia)
Spiders (Arachnophobia)

Diana, Princess of Wales (1 July 1961–31 August 1997)
Thirteen (Number 13) (Triskaidekaphobia)

Diaz, Cameron (30 August 1972–)
Germs (Spermophobia)

Dickens, Charles (7 February 1812–9 June 1870)
Bats (Vespertiliophobia)

Dietrich, Marlene (27 December 1901–6 May 1992)
Germs (Spermophobia)

Disney, Walt (5 December 1901–15 December 1966)
Mice (Musophobia)

Doherty, Shannen (12 April 1971–)
Germs (Spermophobia)

Douglas, Michael (25 September 1945–)
Hair (Excessive Hair) (Hirsutiphobia)

Duff, Hilary (28 September 1987–)
Uncleanliness (Rhypophobia)

Duncan, Isadora (26 May 1877–14 September 1927)
Cars (Autokinetophobia)

Dunst, Kirsten (30 April 1982–)
Flying (Flying in an Aircraft) (Aviophobia)

Dylan, Bob (24 May 1941–)
Social Situations (Sociophobia)

Eastwood, Clint (31 May 1930–)
Horses (Equinophobia)

Edison, Thomas (11 February 1847–18 October 1931)
Public Speaking (Glossophobia)

Einstein, Albert (14 March 1879–18 April 1955)
Social Situations (Sociophobia)

Electra, Carmen (20 April 1972–)
Drowning (Aquaphobia)
Seas (Thalassophobia)

Elizabeth I of England (7 September 1533–24 March 1603)
Flowers (Anthophobia)

Elizabeth, Shannon (7 September 1973–)
Chickens (Alektorophobia)

Eminem (17 October 1972–)
Owls (Ululaphobia)

Estefan, Gloria (1 September 1957–)
Social Situations (Sociophobia)

Ethelred, King (c. 840–23 April 871)
Candles (Candelaphobia)

Farrell, Colin (31 May 1976–)
Flying (Flying in an Aircraft) (Aviophobia)

Feldman, Michael (9 March 1949–)
Social Situations (Sociophobia)

Fellini, Federico (20 January 1920–31 October 1993)
Daylight (Phengophobia)
Noises (Ligyrophobia)

Feydeau, Georges (6 December 1862–5 June 1921)
Daylight (Phengophobia)

Field, Sally (6 November 1946–)
Social Situations (Sociophobia)

Fitzgerald, Ella (25 April 1917–15 June 1996)
Social Situations (Sociophobia)

Fonda, Henry (16 May 1905–12 August 1982)
Social Situations (Sociophobia)

Ford, Harrison (13 July 1942–)
Social Situations (Sociophobia)

Fox, Megan (16 May 1986–)
Flying (Flying in an Aircraft) (Aviophobia)

Fox, Samantha (15 April 1966–)
Snakes (Ophidiophobia)
Spiders (Arachnophobia)

Franklin, Aretha (25 March 1942–)
Flying (Flying in an Aircraft) (Aviophobia)
Public Places (Agoraphobia)

Frederick the Great (24 January 1712–17 August 1786)
Washing (Ablutophobia)
Water (Hydrophobia)

Freud, Sigmund (6 May 1856–23 September 1939)
Plants (Botanophobia)
Trains (Siderodromophobia)
Travel (Hodophobia)

Frost, Robert (26 March 1874–29 January 1963)
Social Situations (Sociophobia)

Garfield, John (4 March 1913–21 May 1952)
Stage (The Stage) (Topophobia)

Gates, Gareth (12 July 1984–)
Bats (Vespertiliophobia)

Gellar, Sarah Michelle (14 April 1977–)
Cemeteries (Coimetrophobia)

Gere, Richard (31 August 1949–)
Dust (Amathophobia)
Social Situations (Sociophobia)

Gest, David (11 May 1953–)
Speaking (Phonophobia)
Telephones (Telephonophobia)

Gibney, Rebecca (14 December 1964–)
Social Situations (Sociophobia)

Goethe, Johann Wolfgang von (28 August 1749–22 March 1832)
Alone (Being Alone) (Eremophobia)
Candles (Candelaphobia)
Darkness (Achluophobia)

Disease (Nosophobia)
Glass (Hyelophobia)
High Places (Acrophobia)
Noises (Ligyrophobia)

Gold, H.L. (26 April 1914–21 February 1996)
Public Places (Agoraphobia)

Goldberg, Whoopi (15 November 1955–)
Flying (Flying in an Aircraft) (Aviophobia)

Goodrem, Delta (9 November 1984–)
Injections (Trypanophobia)

Grable, Betty (18 December 1916–2 July 1973)
Crowds (Ochlophobia)

Graham, Katharine (16 June 1917–17 July 2001)
Social Situations (Sociophobia)

Grahame, Nikki (28 April 1982–)
Meat (Carnophobia)

Grant, Ulysses S. (27 April 1822–23 July 1885)
Social Situations (Sociophobia)

Green, Robson (18 December 1964–)
Wasps (Spheksophobia)

Grint, Rupert (24 August 1988–)
Spiders (Arachnophobia)

Grumman, Leroy (4 January 1895–4 October 1982)
Social Situations (Sociophobia)

Guinness, Alec (2 April 1914–5 August 2000)
Social Situations (Sociophobia)

Hackman, Gene (30 January 1930–)
Social Situations (Sociophobia)

Hamilton, George (12 August 1939–)
Everything (Pantophobia)

Hamm, Mia (17 March 1972–)
Social Situations (Sociophobia)

Hanks, Tom (9 July 1956–)
Social Situations (Sociophobia)

Hannah, Daryl (3 December 1960–)
Public Places (Agoraphobia)

Harriot, Ainsley (28 February 1957–)
Snakes (Ophidiophobia)

Harrison, George (25 February 1943–29 November 2001)
Flying (Flying in an Aircraft) (Aviophobia)
Social Situations (Sociophobia)

Hawthorne, Nathaniel (4 July 1804–19 May 1864)
Social Situations (Sociophobia)

Henderson, Florence (14 February 1934–)
Flying (Flying in an Aircraft) (Aviophobia)

Henry III of France (19 September 1551–2 August 1589)
Cats (Felinophobia)

Hewitt, Jennifer Love (21 February 1979–)
Bogeyman (Bogeyphobia)
Darkness (Achluophobia)
Elevators (Elevatuphobia)
Enclosed Spaces (Claustrophobia)
Sharks (Selachophobia)

Hitchcock, Alfred (13 August 1899–29 April 1980)
Balloons (Pallonophobia)
Cars (Driving a Car) (Mobilophobia)
Eggs (Ovophobia)
Police (Policiphobia)
Smoking (Smykheinophobia)

Hitler, Adolf (20 April 1889–30 April 1945)
Enclosed Spaces (Claustrophobia)

Holt, Kimberly Willis (9 September 1960–)
Social Situations (Sociophobia)

Houdini, Harry (24 March 1874–31 October 1926)
Enclosed Spaces (Claustrophobia)

Howard, Shemp (4 March 1895–22 November 1955)
Cars (Autokinetophobia)
Dogs (Caninophobia)
Flying (Flying in an Aircraft) (Aviophobia)
Water (Hydrophobia)

Hughes, Howard (27 December 1905–5 April 1976)
Germs (Spermophobia)
Public Places (Agoraphobia)

Hussey, Olivia (17 April 1951–)
Public Places (Agoraphobia)

Jackman, Hugh (12 October 1968–)
Dolls (Paediophobia)

Jackson, Glenda (9 May 1936–)
Flying (Flying in an Aircraft) (Aviophobia)

Jackson, Michael (29 August 1958–25 June 2009)
Flying (Flying in an Aircraft) (Aviophobia)
Germs (Spermophobia)

Jagger, Jade (21 October 1971–)
Flying (Flying in an Aircraft) (Aviophobia)

James I of England (19 June 1566–27 March 1625)
Pointed Objects (Aichmophobia)

Jefferson, Thomas (13 April 1743–4 July 1826)
Public Speaking (Glossophobia)

Jelinek, Elfriede (20 October 1946–)
Public Speaking (Glossophobia)
Social Situations (Sociophobia)

Johansson, Scarlett (22 November 1984–)
Cockroaches (Blattaphobia)
Insects (Entomophobia)
Uncleanliness (Rhypophobia)

Johnson, Samuel (18 September 1709–13 December 1784)
Rooms (Koinoniphobia)

Johnstone, Jimmy (30 September 1944–13 March 2006)
Flying (Flying in an Aircraft) (Aviophobia)

Jones, Norah (30 March 1979–)
Clothing (Vestiphobia)
Social Situations (Sociophobia)

Jones, Tommy Lee (15 September 1946–)
Clothing (Vestiphobia)

Jong-il, Kim (16 February 1941–)
Flying (Flying in an Aircraft) (Aviophobia)

Joyce, James (2 February 1882–13 January 1941)
Dogs (Caninophobia)
Thunder (Brontophobia)

Jupitus, Phill (25 June 1962–)
Spiders (Arachnophobia)

Kardashian, Kim (21 October 1980–)
Uncleanliness (Rhypophobia)

Karloff, Boris (23 November 1887–2 February 1969)
Mice (Musophobia)

Keillor, Garrison (7 August 1942–)
Social Situations (Sociophobia)

Kelly, R. (8 January 1967–)
Flying (Flying in an Aircraft) (Aviophobia)

Khan, Ghengis (c. 1162–1227)
Cats (Felinophobia)

Khan, Jemima (30 January 1974–)
Flying (Flying in an Aircraft) (Aviophobia)

Kidman, Nicole (20 June 1967–)
Butterflies (Psychephobia)
Insects (Entomophobia)
Moths (Mottephobia)
Social Situations (Sociophobia)

King, Stephen (21 September 1947–)
High Places (Acrophobia)

Knievel, Evel (7 October 1938–30 November 2007)
Flying (Flying in an Aircraft) (Aviophobia)

Kubrick, Stanley (26 July 1928–7 March 1999)
Flying (Flying in an Aircraft) (Aviophobia)

Lauer, Matt (30 December 1957–)
Vomiting (Emetophobia)

Lenard, Philipp (7 June 1862–20 May 1947)
Names (Nomenatophobia)

Letterman, David (12 April 1947–)
Social Situations (Sociophobia)

Lincoln, Abraham (12 February 1809–15 April 1865)
Dentists (Dentophobia)
Social Situations (Sociophobia)

Longoria, Eva (15 March 1975–)
Injections (Trypanophobia)

Lopez, Jennifer (24 July 1969–)
Darkness (Achluophobia)

Lovett, Lyle (1 November 1957–)
Bulls (Taurophobia)
Cattle (Bovinuphobia)

Lumley, Joanna (1 May 1946–)
Water (Hydrophobia)

Lynn, Loretta (14 April 1935–)
Flying (Flying in an Aircraft) (Aviophobia)

Madden, John (10 April 1936–)
Enclosed Spaces (Claustrophobia)
Flying (Flying in an Aircraft) (Aviophobia)

Madonna (16 August 1958–)
Thunder (Brontophobia)

Maguire, Tobey (27 June 1975–)
High Places (Acrophobia)

Mandell, Howie (29 November 1955–)
Germs (Spermophobia)

Marchand, Nancy (19 June 1928–18 June 2000)
Social Situations (Sociophobia)

Marchant, Amanda (26 June 1988–)
Fish (Icthyophobia)
Sharks (Selachophobia)

Marchant, Samantha (26 June 1988–)
Fish (Icthyophobia)
Sharks (Selachophobia)

Margret, Ann- (28 April 1941–)
Social Situations (Sociophobia)

Marsh, Kym (13 June 1976–)
Flying (Flying in an Aircraft) (Aviophobia)

Martin, Dean (7 June 1917–25 December 1995)
Elevators (Elevatuphobia)
Enclosed Spaces (Claustrophobia)
High Buildings (Batophobia)
High Places (Acrophobia)

McAndrew, Nell (6 November 1973–)
Snakes (Ophidiophobia)
Spiders (Arachnophobia)

McCabe, David (1980–)
Food (Sitophobia)

McCaw, Craig (11 August 1949–)
Social Situations (Sociophobia)

McConaughey, Matthew (4 November 1969–)
Doors (Thuraphobia)
Tunnels (Tubuphobia)

McDonald, Garry (30 October 1948–)
Social Situations (Sociophobia)

McGowan, Rose (5 September 1973–)
Public Places (Agoraphobia)

McGrath, Mark (15 March 1968–)
Elevators (Elevatuphobia)

McLean, Nicola (16 September 1985–)
Butterflies (Psychephobia)
High Places (Acrophobia)
Moths (Mottephobia)
Rats (Rodentophobia)
Snakes (Ophidiophobia)
Spiders (Arachnophobia)

McMahon, Ed (6 March 1923–23 June 2009)
High Places (Acrophobia)

Mears, Charlotte (29 March 1985–)
Balloons (Pallonophobia)

Mirren, Helen (26 July 1945–)
Telephones (Telephonophobia)

Mitchum, Robert (6 August 1917–1 July 1997)
Crowds (Ochlophobia)

Monroe, Marilyn (1 June 1926–5 August 1962)
Public Places (Agoraphobia)

Moore, Roger (14 October 1927–)
Firearms (Hoplophobia)

Murray, Chad Michael (24 August 1981–)
Flying (Flying in an Aircraft) (Aviophobia)

Mussolini, Benito (29 July 1883–28 April 1945)
Cats (Felinophobia)

Myers, Mike (25 May 1965–)
Touched (Being Touched) (Haphephobia)

Navratilova, Martina (18 October 1956–)
Caves (Troglophobia)
High Places (Acrophobia)
Spiders (Arachnophobia)

Neeson, Liam (7 June 1952–)
High Places (Acrophobia)

Newhart, Bob (5 September 1929–)
Flying (Flying in an Aircraft) (Aviophobia)

Oakley, Annie (13 August 1860–3 November 1926)
Social Situations (Sociophobia)

Olivier, Laurence (22 May 1907–11 July 1989)
Stage (The Stage) (Topophobia)

O'Neill, Susie (2 August 1973–)
Social Situations (Sociophobia)

Osbourne, Kelly (27 October 1984–)
Touched (Being Touched) (Haphephobia)

Osmond, Donny (9 December 1957–)
Social Situations (Sociophobia)

Pace, Norman (17 February 1953–)
Reptiles (Herpetophobia)

Pallette, Eugene (8 July 1889–3 September 1954)
Bolshevism (Bolshephobia)

Park, Ray (23 August 1974–)
Insects (Entomophobia)
Spiders (Arachnophobia)

Parker, Sarah Jessica (25 March 1965–)
Flying (Flying in an Aircraft) (Aviophobia)

Pascal, Blaise (19 June 1623–19 August 1662)
Public Places (Agoraphobia)

Pattinson, Robert (13 May 1986–)
Cars (Driving a Car) (Mobilophobia)
Darkness (Achluophobia)

Pfeiffer, Michelle (29 April 1958–)
Drowning (Aquaphobia)
Seas (Thalassophobia)
Social Situations (Sociophobia)

Phoenix, Joaquin (28 October 1974–)
Flying (Flying in an Aircraft) (Aviophobia)

Pitt, Brad (18 December 1963–)
Feet (Podophobia)
Social Situations (Sociophobia)

Poe, Edgar Allan (19 January 1809–7 October 1849)
Buried Alive (Being Buried Alive) (Taphephobia)
Enclosed Spaces (Claustrophobia)

Portman, Natalie (9 June 1981–)
Animated Characters (Animatuphobia)

Potts, Paul (13 October 1970–)
Social Situations (Sociophobia)

Presley, Elvis (8 January 1935–16 August 1977)
Social Situations (Sociophobia)

Prus, Boleslaw (20 August 1847–19 May 1912)
Public Places (Agoraphobia)

Radcliffe, Daniel (23 July 1989–)
Clowns (Coulrophobia)

Rantzen, Esther (22 June 1940–)
Carnivals (Carolevarephobia)
High Places (Acrophobia)
Lavatories (Lavatoriphobia)
Snakes (Ophidiophobia)
Spiders (Arachnophobia)
Water (Hydrophobia)

Reagan, Ronald (6 February 1911–5 June 2004)
Enclosed Spaces (Claustrophobia)
Flying (Flying in an Aircraft) (Aviophobia)

Reeves, Keanu (2 September 1964–)
Darkness (Achluophobia)

Ricci, Christina (12 February 1980–)
Gerbils (Gerbillophobia)

Plants (Botanophobia)
Sharks (Selachophobia)
Spectres (Spectrophobia)
Swimming Pools (Natatoraphobia)

Rice, Anne (4 October 1941–)
Darkness (Achluophobia)

Richard, Wendy (20 July 1943–26 February 2009)
Spiders (Arachnophobia)

Richards, Denise (17 February 1971–)
Vomiting (Emetophobia)

Rickles, Don (8 May 1926–)
Social Situations (Sociophobia)

Rigby, Cathy (12 December 1952–)
Social Situations (Sociophobia)

Rivers, Joan (8 June 1933–)
Social Situations (Sociophobia)

Roberts, Julia (28 October 1967–)
Social Situations (Sociophobia)

Robinson, Peter (aka Marilyn) (3 November 1962–)
Public Places (Agoraphobia)

Rogers, Roy (5 November 1911–6 July 1998)
Social Situations (Sociophobia)

Rooney, Wayne (24 October 1985–)
Flying (Flying in an Aircraft) (Aviophobia)

Roosevelt, Eleanor (11 October 1884–7 November 1962)
Social Situations (Sociophobia)

Roosevelt, Franklin (30 January 1882–12 April 1945)
Thirteen (Number 13) (Triskaidekaphobia)

Roosevelt, Theodore (28 October 1858–6 January 1919)
Social Situations (Sociophobia)

Rossini, Gioachino (29 February 1792–13 November 1868)
Friday the 13th (Paraskavedekatriaphobia)

Russo, Rene (17 February 1954–)
Social Situations (Sociophobia)

Ryan, Justin (11 February 1966–)
Insects (Entomophobia)

Sartre, Jean-Paul (21 June 1905–15 April 1980)
Shellfish (Ostraconophobia)

Schiller, Johann Christoph Friedrich von
(10 November 1750–9 May 1805)
Spiders (Arachnophobia)

Schopenhauer, Arthur (22 February 1788–21 September 1860)
Barbers (Barbaphobia)
Fire (Pyrophobia)

Schumann, Robert (8 June 1810–29 July 1856)
Metal (Metallophobia)

Schuur, Diane (10 December 1953–)
Social Situations (Sociophobia)

Shakira (2 February 1977–)
Death (Thanatophobia)

Shalit, Gene (25 March 1932–)
Flying (Flying in an Aircraft) (Aviophobia)

Shaw, George Bernard (26 July 1856–2 November 1950)
Social Situations (Sociophobia)

Siversen, Louise (25 May 1960–)
Social Situations (Sociophobia)

Smith, Robert (21 April 1959–)
Flying (Flying in an Aircraft) (Aviophobia)

Sonnenfeld, Barry (1 April 1953–)
Flying (Flying in an Aircraft) (Aviophobia)

Spears, Britney (2 December 1981–)
Reptiles (Herpetophobia)

Spielberg, Steven (18 December 1946–)
Insects (Entomophobia)

Steinberg, David (9 August 1942–)
Snakes (Ophidiophobia)

Stevens, Rachel (9 April 1978–)
Lavatories (Lavatoriphobia)

Stiles, Ryan (22 April 1959–)
Flying (Flying in an Aircraft) (Aviophobia)

Stone, Sharon (10 March 1958–)
Television (TV-phobia)

Stowe, Harriet Beecher (14 June 1811–1 July 1896)
Social Situations (Sociophobia)

Streisand, Barbra (24 April 1942–)
Human Beings (Anthropophobia)

Swash, Joe (20 January 1982–)
Rats (Rodentophobia)
Snakes (Ophidiophobia)

Thornton, Billy Bob (4 August 1955–)
Antiques (Antiquphobia)
Colours (Chromophobia)
Flying (Flying in an Aircraft) (Aviophobia)

Thurman, Uma (29 April 1970–)
Enclosed Spaces (Claustrophobia)

Timberlake, Justin (31 January 1981–)
Sharks (Selachophobia)
Snakes (Ophidiophobia)
Spiders (Arachnophobia)

Trump, Donald (14 June 1946–)
Germs (Spermophobia)

Tureaud, Laurence "Mr T" (21 May 1952–)
Flying (Flying in an Aircraft) (Aviophobia)

Underwood, Carrie (10 March 1983–)
Social Situations (Sociophobia)

Valance, Holly (11 May 1983–)
Flying (Flying in an Aircraft) (Aviophobia)

Von Trier, Lars (30 April 1956–)
Flying (Flying in an Aircraft) (Aviophobia)

Warhol, Andy (6 August 1928–22 February 1987)
Hospitals (Nosocomephobia)

Washington, Sabrina (27 October 1978–)
Flying (Flying in an Aircraft) (Aviophobia)
High Places (Acrophobia)

Weaver, Sigourney (8 October 1949–)
Social Situations (Sociophobia)

Webbe, Simon (30 March 1978–)
Everything (Pantophobia)

White, Jimmy (2 May 1962–)
Snakes (Ophidiophobia)

Wilson, Brian (20 June 1942–)
Public Places (Agoraphobia)

Winfrey, Oprah (29 January 1954–)
Chewing Gum (Mastichegummiphobia)

Wood, Natalie (20 July 1938–29 November 1981)
Drowning (Aquaphobia)

Woodburn, Kim (25 March 1942–)
Insects (Entomophobia)

Woodward, Joanne (27 February 1930–)
Flying (Flying in an Aircraft) (Aviophobia)

Woolf, Virginia (25 January 1882–28 March 1941)
Pictures (Pictophobia)

Wright, Ian (17 May 1965–)
Enclosed Spaces (Claustrophobia)

Wright, Orville (19 August 1871–30 January 1948)
Social Situations (Sociophobia)

Zucker, Carly (11 May 1984–)
Insects (Entomophobia)
Snakes (Ophidiophobia)

Chapter 24
Phobia Names

"To fear love is to fear life, and those who fear life are already three parts dead."

Bertrand Russell (1872–1970), *Marriage and Morals*

Each phobia name and its source are listed below.

ABANNUMAPHOBIA — Abandonment

ABLUTOPHOBIA — Washing

ABORTIVUPHOBIA — Abortion

ACAROPHOBIA — Mites

ACCULTURAPHOBIA — Acculturation

ACEROPHOBIA — Sourness

ACHLUOPHOBIA — Darkness

ACIDUSRIGAREPHOBIA — Acid Rain

ACONSCIUSIOPHOBIA — Unconsciousness

ACOUSTICOPHOBIA — Sounds

ACROPHOBIA — High Places

ACROTOMOPHOBIA — Amputees

ACUSAPUNGEREPHOBIA — Acupuncture

ADDICEROPHOBIA — Addiction

AEROACROPHOBIA — Open High Places

AEROEMPHYSEMAPHOBIA — Bends (The Bends)

AERONAUSIPHOBIA — Air Sickness

AEROPHOBIA — Air

AEROPOLLUEREPHOBIA — Air Pollution

AESOPHOBIA — Brass

AETATEMOPHOBIA — Aging

AFROPHOBIA — Africa (Things African)

AGONOPHOBIA — Rape (Pretended Rape)

AGONOSOPHOBIA — Unknown (The Unknown)

AGORAPHOBIA — Public Places

AGRAPHOBIA — Abuse

AGREXOPHOIA — Love (Making Love)

AGRIZOOPHOBIA — Animals (Wild)

AIBOPHOBIA — Palindromes

AICHMOPHOBIA — Pointed Objects

AIDS-PHOBIA — AIDS

AKLYOPHOBIA — Deafness

ALBUMINUROPHOBIA — Kidney Diseases

ALEKTOROPHOBIA — Chickens

ALGOPHOBIA — Pain (One's Own)

ALKEPHOBIA — Deer

ALLIUMPHOBIA — Garlic

ALLODOXAPHOBIA — Opposing Opinions

ALTOCALCIPHOBIA — Boots

AMARUPHOBIA — Bitterness

AMATHOPHOBIA — Dust

AMAUROPHOBIA — Blindness (Being or Becoming Blind)

AMAXOPHOBIA — Carriages

AMBULAPHOBIA — Body Movement

AMERIPHOBIA — America (Things American)

AMNESIOPHOBIA — Amnesia

AMYCHOPHOBIA — Scratched (Being Scratched)

ANABLEPOPHOBIA — Looking Up

ANASTEEMAPHOBIA — Height Differences

ANDROGYNOPHOBIA — Masking Gender

ANDROMIMETOPHOBIA — Females Imitating Males

ANDROPHOBIA — Men

ANDROTIKOLOBOMASSOPHOBIA — Ears (Ears of a Male)

ANECOPHOBIA — Homelessness

ANEMOPHOBIA — Wind

ANGINOPHOBIA — Narrowness

ANGLOPHOBIA — England (Things English)

ANGROPHOBIA — Anger

ANIMATUPHOBIA — Animated Characters

ANKYLOPHOBIA — Joint Immobility

ANTHOPHOBIA — Flowers

ANTHROPOPHOBIA — Human Beings

ANTIQUPHOBIA — Antiques

ANTLOPHOBIA — Floods

ANUPTAPHOBIA — Unmarried (Being Unmarried)

APEIROPHOBIA — Infinity

APHRONEMOPHOBIA — Thinking (Irrational)

APOCALYPSIPHOBIA — Apocalypse (The Apocalypse)

APOTEMNOPHOBIA — Amputations

APPROBAREPHOBIA — Approval

AQUAPHOBIA — Drowning

ARACHIBUTYROPHOBIA — Peanut Butter

ARACHNOPHOBIA — Spiders

ARCANOPHOBIA — Magic

ARCHTOPHOBIA — Teddy Bears

ARCUSAPHOBIA — Arches

ARGENTUPHOBIA — Silver

ARHYPOPHOBIA — Cleanliness

ARSONPHOBIA — Arson

ASCENDAREPHOBIA — Climbing

ASIAPHOBIA — Asia (Things Asian)

ASPHYXIOPHOBIA — Self-strangulation

ASTHENOPHOBIA — Weakness

ASTRAPHOBIA — Celestial Space

ASTROLOGIAPHOBIA — Astrology

ASYMMETRIPHOBIA — Asymmetry

ATANPHOBIA — Oats

ATAXIAPHOBIA — Ataxia

ATAXIOPHOBIA — Disorder

ATELOPHOBIA — Imperfection

ATEPHOBIA — Ruin (Being Ruined)

ATHAZAGORAPHOBIA — Forgotten (Being Forgotten)

ATOMOSOPHOBIA — Atomic Energy and Science

ATYCHIPHOBIA — Defeat

AUCTORITAPHOBIA — Authority

AULOPHOBIA — Wind Instruments

AURANJAPHOBIA — Orange (Colour or Word)

AUROPHOBIA — Gold

AURORAPHOBIA — Auroras

AUSTRALOPHOBIA — Australia (Things Australian)

AUTAGONISTOPHOBIA — Cameras (Appearing on Camera)

AUTISM-PHOBIA — Autism

AUTOASSASSINOPHOBIA — Murder (One's Own)

AUTODYSOMOPHOBIA — Body Odour (One's Own)

AUTOKINETOPHOBIA — Cars

AUTOMATONOPHOBIA — Animatronic Creatures

AUTOMYSOPHOBIA — Body Dirt (One's Own)

AUTOPHOBIA — Self (The Self)

AVIDSOPHOBIA — Bird (Being or Becoming a Bird)

AVIOPHOBIA — Flying (Flying in an Aircraft)

BACILLOPHOBIA — Bacilli

BACTERIOPHOBIA — Bacteria

BALLISTOPHOBIA — Bullets

BANANAPHOBIA — Bananas

BARBAPHOBIA — Barbers

BARLEYPHOBIA — Barley

BAROPHOBIA — Gravity

BASIOPHOBIA — Walking

BATHMOPHOBIA — Thresholds

BATHOPHOBIA — Depths

BATHYSIDERODROMOPHOBIA — Subways

BATOPHOBIA — High Buildings

BATRACHOPHOBIA — Amphibians (Anything Amphibious)

BATTUEREPHOBIA — Beating Oneself

BELLUMAPHOBIA — War

BELLUSAPHOBIA — Beauty Salons

BELONOPHOBIA — Needles

BIASTOPHOBIA — Sexual Assault

BIBLIOPHOBIA — Books

BINIPHOBIA — Twins

BLAIREAUPHOBIA — Badgers

BLATTAPHOBIA — Cockroaches

BLENNOPHOBIA — Mucus

BOEIPHOBIA — Boys

BOGEYPHOBIA — Bogeyman

BOLSHEPHOBIA — Bolshevism

BORBORYGAMIPHOBIA — Stomach Gurgling

BOTANOPHOBIA — Plants

BOTTIAPHOBIA — Buttons

BOVINUPHOBIA — Cattle

BREKHMOPHOBIA — Brain

BROMIDROSIPHOBIA — Body Odour Embarrassment (Another's)

BRONTOPHOBIA — Thunder

BROUNPHOBIA — Brown (Colour or Word)

BRUNDISIPHOBIA — Bronze

BUDDHISTOPHOBIA — Buddhism

BUFONOPHOBIA — Toads

CACOPHOBIA — Ugliness

CAD-PHOBIA — Coronary Artery Disease

CADENTEMOPHOBIA — Gambling

CALIANDROPHOBIA — Beautiful Men (Handsome Men)

CALIGYNEPHOBIA — Beautiful Women (Handsome Women)

CANINOPHOBIA — Dogs

CANNABIPHOBIA — Cannabis

CAPITALIPHOBIA — Capitalism

CARBOHYDRAPHOBIA — Carbohydrates

CARCINOMATOPHOBIA — Cancer

CARDIACHIRURGIAPHOBIA — Heart Surgery

CARDIOPATHOPHOBIA — Heart Disease

CARDIOPHOBIA — Heart

CARNOPHOBIA — Meat

CAROLEVAREPHOBIA — Carnivals

CASICAREPHOBIA — Waterfalls

CASTRATAPHOBIA — Castration

CATAGELOPHOBIA — Ridicule

CATAPEDAPHOBIA — Jumping

CATARACTAPHOBIA — Cataracts

CATHISOPHOBIA — Sitting

CATHOLICOPHOBIA — Catholicism

CDLD-PHOBIA — Coal Dust Lung Disease

CELTOPHOBIA — Celts (Things Celtic)

CETUSAPHOBIA — Marine Mammals

CFS-PHOBIA — Chronic Fatigue Syndrome

CHAOSOPHOBIA — Chaos

CHEIMAPHOBIA — Cold (Cold Things)

CHELONAPHOBIA — Turtles

CHEMOPHOBIA — Chemicals

CHEMOTHERAPIEPHOBIA — Chemotherapy

CHEROPHOBIA — Happiness (Being Happy)

CHF-PHOBIA — Congestive Heart Failure

CHIONOPHOBIA — Snow

CHIROPHOBIA — Hands

CHLAMYDIA-PHOBIA — Chlamydia

CHLOROPHOBIA — Green (Colour or Word)

CHOLERAPHOBIA — Cholera

CHOLEROPHOBIA — Anger (Another's)

CHOLESTEROPHOBIA — Cholesterol

CHOROPHOBIA — Dancing

CHREMATISTOPHOBIA — Robbed (Being Robbed)

CHREMATOPHOBIA — Money

CHRIMATOPHOBIA — Finances

CHRISTOPHOBIA — Christianity

CHROMOANTHROPOPHOBIA — Coloured People (People of
Colour)

CHROMOPHOBIA — Colours

CHRONOMENTROPHOBIA — Clocks

CHRONOPHOBIA — Time

CHRONOSPOINEPHOBIA — Chronic Pain

CLAUDEREPHOBIA — Fences

CLAUSTROPHOBIA — Enclosed Spaces

CLIMACOPHOBIA — Stairs

CLIMATEPHOBIA — Climate

CLINOPHOBIA — Beds

CNIDOPHOBIA — Stingers

COCAINE-PHOBIA — Cocaine

COIMETROPHOBIA — Cemeteries

COITOPHOBIA — Coitus

COITUSINTERCURSUPHOBIA — Sexual Intercourse

COITUSMOREFERAPHOBIA — Sexual Contact Involving Wild Beasts

COITUSORALISIPHOBIA — Sexual Contact Involving the Mouth

COMETOPHOBIA — Comets

COMMITMENTPHOBIA — Commitment

COMMUNISMPHOBIA — Communism

COMPETERAPHOBIA — Competition

COMPUTERPHOBIA — Computers

CONDOMOPHOBIA — Condoms

CONFRONTAPHOBIA — Confrontation

CONSCIUSIOPHOBIA — Consciousness

CONSECOTALEOPHOBIA — Chopsticks

CONTINGEREPHOBIA — Contagious (Being Contagious)

CONTRAROTAPHOBIA — Control

CONTRECTOPHOBIA — Sexual Abuse

COPD-PHOBIA — Chronic Obstructive Pulmonary Disease

COPRASTASOPHOBIA — Constipation

COPROPHOBIA — Faeces

CORNUAPHOBIA — Corners

CORNUPHOBIA — Corn

CORONAPHOBIA — Crowns

COULROPHOBIA — Clowns

COUNTERPHOBIA — Fear Avoidance

CREATUSIPHOBIA — Creativity

CREMNOPHOBIA — Cliffs

CRONOPHOBIA — Time

CRYOPHOBIA — Cold (Extreme Cold)

CRYSTALLOPHOBIA — Crystals

CTS-PHOBIA — Carpal Tunnel Syndrome

CULTUSOPHOBIA — Cults

CURSUSOPHOBIA — Curses

CYANOPHOBIA — Blue (Colour or Word)

CYBERPHOBIA — Cyberspace

CYCLOANEMOPHOBIA — Cyclones

CYCLOPHOBIA — Bicycles

CYPRIDOPHOBIA — Prostitutes

CYPRIPHOBIA — Sexually Transmitted Diseases

DACRYPHOBIA — Tears

DACTYLOPHOBIA — Fingers

DACTYLOPUNGEREPHOBIA — Finger Pointing

DARATAPHOBIA — Wheat

DATUSIOPHOBIA — Dating

DECAPITAPHOBIA — Decapitation (Being Decapitated)

DECIDOPHOBIA — Decisions (Making Decisions)

DEFECALGESIOPHOBIA — Bowel Movements

DEFECTUPHOBIA — Defects

DEIPNOPHOBIA — Dining

DELUDEREPHOBIA — Delusions

DEMENTOPHOBIA — Dementia

DEMONOPHOBIA — Demons

DENDROPHOBIA — Trees

DENTOPHOBIA — Dentists

DEPRESSAREPHOBIA— Depression

DERMATOPATHOPHOBIA — Skin Disease

DERMATOPHOBIA — Skin

DESERTPHOBIA — Deserts

DESYNCHRONOPHOBIA — Jet Lag

DEVORAPHOBIA — Eaten (Being Eaten)

DEXTROPHOBIA — Right-handedness

DIABETOPHOBIA — Diabetes

DIARRHOEAPHOBIA — Diarrhoea

DIESOMNIUPHOBIA — Daydreaming

DIET-PHOBIA — Dieting

DIKEPHOBIA — Justice

DINOPHOBIA — Whirlpools

DIPLOPHOBIA — Double Vision

DIPSOPHOBIA — Drinking

DISHABILIOPHOBIA — Undressing

DIVORTIPHOBIA — Divorce

DOMATOPHOBIA — House (Being in a House)

DORAPHOBIA — Animal Skins and Fur

DOXOPHOBIA — Opinions

DROMOPHOBIA — Streets

DUTCHPHOBIA — Dutch (The Dutch)

DYSMORPHOPHOBIA — Deformity

DYSOMOPHOBIA — Body Odour (Another's)

DYSPHOPHOBIA — Bad News

DYSTYCHIPHOBIA — Accidents

ECCLESIOPHOBIA — Churches

ECDYSIAPHOBIA — Strippers

ECOPHOBIA — Home

EDIFICIPHOBIA — Buildings

EISODOPHOBIA — Virginity

EISOPTROPHOBIA — Mirrors

EJACULAPHOBIA — Ejaculation

ELECTROCONVULSIPHOBIA — Electroconvulsive Therapy

ELECTROPHOBIA — Electricity

ELEUTHEROPHOBIA — Freedom

ELEVATUPHOBIA — Elevators

EMETOPHOBIA — Vomiting

ENDYTOPHOBIA — Dressing

ENETOPHOBIA — Pins

ENEURESISSOPHOBIA — Bed-wetting

ENISSOPHOBIA — Reproach

ENTOMOPHOBIA — Insects

EOSOPHOBIA — Dawn

EPHEBOPHOBIA — Adolescent Males

EPILEPSY-PHOBIA — Epilepsy

EPISTAXIOPHOBIA — Nosebleeds

EPISTEMOPHOBIA — Knowledge

EPISTOLOPHOBIA — Letters

EQINOPHOBIA — Horses

EREMOPHOBIA — Alone (Being Alone)

EREUTHROPHOBIA — Red (Colour or Word)

ERGASIOPHOBIA — Work

EROTOPHOBIA — Eroticism

ERUCTAPHOBIA — Belching

ERYTHROPHOBIA — Blushing

ETERNALIPHOBIA — Eternity

EUPHOPHOBIA — Good News

EUROPOPHOBIA — Europe (Things European)

EUROTOPHOBIA — Vaginas

EXAMINAPHOBIA — Examinations (Academic)

EXERCISE-PHOBIA — Exercise

FABRICAPHOBIA — Fabrics (Specific)

FAERIOPHOBIA — Faeries

FASCISMPHOBIA — Fascism

FEBRIPHOBIA — Fever

FELINOPHOBIA — Cats

FERRUMPHOBIA — Iron

FISSURAPHOBIA — Fissures

FLATULENTIAPHOBIA — Flatulence

FORAREPHOBIA — Boredom

FORISOPOMOPHOBIA — Doorknobs

FORMICOPHOBIA — Ants

FRANCOPHOBIA — France (Things French)
FRIEND-OR-PHOBIA — Passwords
FRUSTRATUPHOBIA — Frustration

GALEOPHOBIA — Weasels
GAMOPHOBIA — Marriage
GASTROENTERIKOPHOBIA — Gastrointestinal Complaints
GELIOPHOBIA — Laughter (One's Own)
GENIOPHOBIA — Chins
GENOPHOBIA — Sex
GENUPHOBIA — Knees
GENVERRUCAPHOBIA — Genital Warts
GEPHYROPHOBIA — Bridges
GERASCOPHOBIA — Elderly (Being Elderly)
GERBILLOPHOBIA — Gerbils
GERMANOPHOBIA — Germany (Things German)
GERONTOPHOBIA — Elderly People
GEUMAPHOBIA — Taste
GLOBAL WARMING-PHOBIA — Global Warming
GLOBAPHOBIA — Globalisation
GLOSSOPHOBIA — Public Speaking
GLUTTONOPHOBIA — Overeating
GNOSOPHOBIA — Known (The Known)
GONORRHOIAPHOBIA — Gonorrhoea
GONYPHOBIA — Knee Bending Backwards
GRAPHOPHOBIA — Handwriting
GRAVAREPHOBIA — Bereavement
GROSSUSOPHOBIA — Big Objects and Things
GULOPHOBIA — Wolverines
GYMNOPHOBIA — Nudity
GYNEMIMETOPHOBIA — Males Imitating Females
GYNEPHOBIA — Women

GYNOTIKOLOBOMASSOPHOBIA — Ears (Ears of a Female)

HABITUSIOPHOBIA — Habits

HADEPHOBIA — Hell

HAEMATOPHOBIA — Blood

HAEMORRHOIDAEPHOBIA — Haemorrhoids

HAGIOPHOBIA — Holy Things

HALITOPHOBIA — Bad Breath

HALLUCINATUPHOBIA — Hallucinations

HALOPHOBIA — Breath

HAMARTOPHOBIA — Errors

HAPHEPHOBIA — Touched (Being Touched)

HARPAXOPHOBIA — Robbing

HEBEPHOBIA — Teenagers

HEDONOPHOBIA — Pleasure

HELIOPHOBIA — Sun (The Sun)

HELLENOLOGOPHOBIA — Scientific Terms

HELLENOPHOBIA — Greece (Things Greek)

HELMINTHOPHOBIA — Worms

HEMICRANIAPHOBIA — Headaches

HEPATITIS-PHOBIA — Hepatitis

HEREIOPHOBIA — Heresy

HERPETOPHOBIA — Reptiles

HETEROPHOBIA — Heterosexuality

HEXAKOSIOIHEXEKONTAHEXAPHOBIA — Six Hundred and Sixty-six (Number 666)

HIEROPHOBIA — Religious Objects

HINDUISTOPHOBIA — Hinduism

HIRSUTIPHOBIA — Hair (Excessive Hair)

HODOPHOBIA — Travel

HOMICHLOPHOBIA — Fog

HOMILOPHOBIA — Sermons

HOMOCIDEPHOBIA — Murder (Another's)

HOMOPHOBIA — Homosexuality

HOPLOPHOBIA — Firearms

HORMEPHOBIA — Shock

HSV-PHOBIA — Herpes Simplex Virus

HYBRISTOPHOBIA — Criminals

HYDRARGYROPHOBIA — Medicines (Mercurial)

HYDROPHOBIA — Water

HYELOEPISTEGOPHOBIA — Glass Ceilings

HYELOPHOBIA — Glass

HYGROPHOBIA — Body Fluids

HYLEPHOBIA — Materialism

HYLOPHOBIA — Forests

HYPENGYOPHOBIA — Responsibility

HYPERTHYROID-PHOBIA — Hyperthyroidism

HYPERTRICHOPHOBIA — Hair ("Bad" Hair)

HYPHEPHOBIA — Fabrics (Non-clothing)

HYPNOPHOBIA — Hypnosis

HYPOGLYCAEMIAPHOBIA — Hypoglycaemia

HYSTERECTOMOPHOBIA — Hysterectomy

HYSTERIKOPHOBIA — Hysteria

IATROPHOBIA — Doctors

IBS-PHOBIA — Irritable Bowel Syndrome

ICONOPHOBIA — Icons

ICTHYOLAKKOPHOBIA — Fish Tanks

ICTHYOPHOBIA — Fish

IDEOPHOBIA — Ideas

ILLYNGOPHOBIA — Dizziness

IMPOTENTOPHOBIA — Impotence

INANIREPHOBIA — Starvation

INCESTUPHOBIA — Incest

INCONTINEPHOBIA — Urinary Incontinence

INDIAPHOBIA — India (Things Indian)

INDIGESTIOPHOBIA — Indigestion

INFANTIPHOBIA — Infants

INFERTILIPHOBIA — Infertility

INSOMNIAPHOBIA — Insomnia

INSULAPHOBIA — Islands

INVIDIAPHOBIA — Envy

IOPHOBIA — Rust

IRISOPHOBIA — Rainbows

ISLAMOPHOBIA — Islam

ISLANDOPHOBIA — Iceland

ISOPTEROPHOBIA — Termites

ITALOPHOBIA — Italy (Things Italian)

JAPONOPHOBIA — Japan (Things Japanese)

JUDAEOPHOBIA — Judaism

KENOPHOBIA — Barren Spaces

KERAUNOPHOBIA — Lightning

KINESOPHOBIA — Movement

KLEPTOPHOBIA — Stealing

KLISMAPHOBIA — Enemas

KLYOPHOBIA — Listening

KOINONIPHOBIA — Rooms

KOPOPHOBIA — Fatigue

KOSMOPHOBIA — Cosmos

KRITIKOPHOBIA — Criticism

KYMOPHOBIA — Waves

KYPHOPHOBIA — Stooping

LACHANOPHOBIA — Vegetables

LACTAPHOBIA — Breast-feeding

LACTOPHOBIA — Milk

LAGOPHOBIA — Rabbits

LARYNGOXEROPHOBIA — Dry Throat

LATEXOPHOBIA — Latex

LAVATORIPHOBIA — Lavatories

LEMUREPHOBIA — Vampires

LENTUPHOBIA — Slowness

LEONTOPHOBIA — Lions

LEOPARDOSOPHOBIA — Leopards

LEPROPHOBIA — Leprosy

LEUKOPHOBIA — White (Colour or Word)

LEVISIPHOBIA — Floating

LIBROPHOBIA — Balance (Being Balanced)

LIGYROPHOBIA — Noises

LILAPSOPHOBIA — Violent Storms

LIMNOPHOBIA — Lakes

LINGERIEPHOBIA — Lingerie

LINONOPHOBIA — String

LITICAPHOBIA — Legal Proceedings

LOBOTOMOPHOBIA — Lobotomy

LOCUSAPHOBIA — Places (Specific Places)

LOGOPHOBIA — Words

LUNAPHOBIA — Moon (The Moon)

LUTRAPHOBIA — Furry Aquatic Animals

LYCANTHROPOPHOBIA — Wolves

LYGOPHOBIA — Gloom

LYSSOPHOBIA — Insanity (One's Own)

LYSUSEISODOPHOBIA — Losing One's Virginity

MACROPHOBIA — Waiting

MAGEIROCOPHOBIA — Cooking

MAIEUSIOPHOBIA — Pregnancy

MAMMAGYMNOPHOBIA — Breasts (Female)

MAMMANDROPHOBIA — Breasts (Male)

MAMMAPHOBIA — Breasts

MANIAPHOBIA — Insanity (Another's)

MARXOPHOBIA — Marxism

MASERPHOBIA — Singapore (Things Singaporean)

MASTICHEGUMMIPHOBIA — Chewing Gum

MASTIGOPHOBIA — Beaten in Public (Being Beaten in Public)

MATERAPHOBIA — Mothers

MECHANOPHOBIA — Machines

MEDOMALACUPHOBIA — Erectile Dysfunction

MEDORTHOPHOBIA— Penises (Erect)

MEGABIOPHOBIA — Large Animals

MEGALOPHOBIA — Large Objects and Things

MELANOPHOBIA — Black (Colour or Word)

MELCRYTOVESTIMENTAPHOBIA — Black Underwear

MELISSAPHOBIA — Bees

MELOPHOBIA — Music

MENDICAREPHOBIA — Beggars

MENINGITOPHOBIA — Brain Disease

MENOPAUSEPHOBIA — Menopause

MENOPHOBIA — Menstruation

MENTALISRETARDEPHOBIA — Disability (Intellectual)

MERCURIOPHOBIA — Mercury

MERINTHOPHOBIA — Bound (Being Bound)

METALLOPHOBIA — Metal

METATHESIOPHOBIA — Beyond (The Beyond)

METEOROPHOBIA — Meteors

METHYLPHOBIA — Alcohol

METROPHOBIA — Poetry

MICROBIOPHOBIA — Small Animals

MICROPHOBIA — Small Objects and Things

MINIMALPHOBIA — Minimalism

MNEMOPHOBIA — Memory (Memories)

MOBILOPHOBIA — Cars (Driving a Car)

MOLYSMOPHOBIA — Infection

MONITORPHOBIA — Monitored (Being Monitored)

MONOPHOBIA — One Thing

MORPHOHYGROPHOBIA — Damp Things

MOTORPHOBIA — Cars (Being a Passenger in a Car)

MOTTEPHOBIA — Moths

MPV-PHOBIA — Mitral Valve Prolapse

MUSEUMOPHOBIA — Museums

MUSOPHOBIA — Mice

MYCOPHOBIA — Mushrooms

MYSOPHOBIA — Body Dirt (Another's)

MYTHOPHOBIA — Myths

NANOSOPHOBIA — Dwarfs

NARCOLEPSIPHOBIA — Narcolepsy

NARRATOPHOBIA — Pornographic Texts

NASOPHOBIA — Noses

NATALISOPHOBIA — Birthdays

NATATORAPHOBIA — Swimming Pools

NAUSEAPHOBIA — Nausea

NAUTOPHOBIA — Ships

NAZISMPHOBIA — Nazism

NECROPHOBIA — Corpses

NEGROFELINOPHOBIA — Black Cats

NEGROPHOBIA — Black People

NEOPHARMACOPHOBIA — Medicines (New)

NEOPHOBIA — New (Anything New)

NEPHOPHOBIA — Clouds

NILHILOPHOBIA — Nothing

NOCENTEMOPHOBIA — Guilt

NOCEREPHOBIA — Nuisances

NOMENATOPHOBIA — Names

NORMOPHOBIA — Conformity

NORTH AMEROPHOBIA — North America (Things North American)

NOSOCOMEPHOBIA — Hospitals

NOSOPHOBIA — Disease

NOSTOPHOBIA — Home (Returning Home)

NOVERCAPHOBIA — Stepmothers

NUMEROPHOBIA — Numbers

NYCTOHYLOPHOBIA — Forests at Night

NYCTOPHOBIA — Night

NYMPHOPHOBIA — Adolescent Females

OBESOPHOBIA — Obesity

OBLIGATIOPHOBIA — Obligations

OBLIVIOPHOBIA — Oblivion

OBSESSIOPHOBIA — Obsessions

OCD-PHOBIA — Obsessive-Compulsive Disorder

OCHLOPHOBIA — Crowds

OCHOPHOBIA — Moving Vehicle (Being in a Moving Vehicle)

OCTOPHOBIA — Eight (Number Eight)

OCULOPHOBIA — Eyes

ODONTOACHOPHOBIA — Toothaches

ODONTOPHOBIA — Teeth

OENOPHOBIA — Wine

OLFACTOPHOBIA — Odours (Certain)

OMBROPHOBIA — Rain (Being Rained On)

OMMATOMALAPHOBIA — Evil Eye

OMNIBUSOPHOBIA — Buses

ONEIROGMOPHOBIA — Wet Dreams

ONEIROPHOBIA — Dreams

ONOMATOPHOBIA — Named (Being Named)

ONYCHOPHOBIA — Nails (Fingers and Toes)

OPHIDIOPHOBIA — Snakes

OPIOPHOBIA — Medicines (Prescription)

OPTAREPHOBIA — Shopping

OPTOPHOBIA — Eyes (Opening One's Eyes)

ORALISIPHOBIA — Mouth

ORCHIDOPHOBIA — Orchids

ORDINEMOPHOBIA — Order

ORNITHOPHOBIA — Birds

ORTHOPHOBIA — Propriety

ORTOGRAPHOBIA — Spelling Mistakes

ORYZAPHOBIA — Rice

OSPHRESIOPHOBIA — Body Odour Embarrassment (One's Own)

OSTRACONOPHOBIA — Shellfish

OTOXEROPHOBIA — Dry Mouth

OVOPHOBIA — Eggs

PAEDIOPHOBIA — Dolls

PAEDOPHOBIA — Children

PAGOPHOBIA — Frost

PALLONOPHOBIA — Balloons

PANICOPHOBIA — Panic

PANPHOBIA — All Things

PANTHER-PHOBIA — Panthers

PANTOPHOBIA — Everything

PAPAPHOBIA — Popes

PAPYROPHOBIA — Paper

PARADOXOPHOBIA — Paradoxes

PARALIPOPHOBIA — Neglect of Duty

PARAMNESIAPHOBIA — Déjà Vu

PARANOIAPHOBIA — Paranoia

PARAPHOBIA — Sexual Perversions

PARAPLEGAPHOBIA — Disability (Physical)

PARASITIOPHOBIA — Parasites

PARASKAVEDEKATRIAPHOBIA — Friday the 13th

PARENTEPHOBIA — Parents

PARTHENOPHOBIA — Girls

PARTURIPHOBIA — Labour (Being in Labour)

PATEROPHOBIA — Fathers

PATHOPHOBIA — Suffering

PATRIOPHOBIA — Heredity

PECCATOPHOBIA — Sin

PEDICOOPERIPHOBIA — Shoes

PELADOPHOBIA — Bald People

PELLAGRAPHOBIA — Pellagra

PENIAPHOBIA — Poverty (One's Own)

PENNAPHOBIA — Wings

PENTHERAPHOBIA — Mothers-in-law

PENTHEROPHOBIA — Fathers-in-law

PERFECTUPHOBIA — Perfection

PERSONALIPARENTOPHOBIA — Parenting

PHAGOPHOBIA — Eating Uncontrollably

PHALACROPHOBIA — Bald (Being or Becoming Bald)

PHALLOPHOBIA — Penises (Non-erect)

PHANTASICOMPANIOPHOBIA — Imaginary Companions

PHARMACOPHOBIA — Medicines

PHENGOPHOBIA — Daylight

PHILEMAPHOBIA — Kissing

PHILOPHOBIA — Love (Being in Love)

PHILOSOPHOBIA — Philosophy

PHOBOPHOBIA — Fears

PHOBOPHOBIAPHOBIA — Fear of Fear of Phobias

PHONOPHOBIA — Speaking

PHOTOALGIAPHOBIA — Eye Pain

PHOTOAUGLIAPHOBIA — Lights (Glaring Lights)

PHOTOBOLBOSOPHOBIA — Light Bulbs

PHOTOPHOBIA — Light

PHRENOPHOBIA — Mental Illness

PHRONEMOPHOBIA — Thinking (Rational)

PHTHEIROPHOBIA — Lice

PHYGEPHOBIA — Chased (Being Chased)

PICTOPHOBIA — Pictures

PINGUIPHOBIA — Fat

PIPAREPHOBIA — Pipes (Solid)

PLACOPHOBIA — Tombstones

PLAGAPHOBIA — Plague

PLANNUMAPHOBIA — Plans (Definite Plans)

PLEGEPHOBIA — Stroke

PLEURODELIPHOBIA — Newts

PLS-PHOBIA — Phantom Limb Syndrome

PLUMBISMUPHOBIA — Lead Poisoning

PLUTOPHOBIA — Wealth

PLUVIOPHOBIA — Showers (Taking a Shower)

PMS-PHOBIA — Premenstrual Syndrome

PND-PHOBIA — Postnatal Depression

PNEUMATOPHOBIA — Spritual Things

PNIGEROPHOBIA — Smothering (Being Smothered)

PNIGOPHOBIA — Choking (Being Choked)

PODOPHOBIA — Feet

POGONOPHOBIA — Beards

POINEPHOBIA — Punishment (Punishment in All Forms)

POLICIOPHOBIA — Police

POLIOSOPHOBIA — Polio

POLITICOPHOBIA — Government

POLLUTIOPHOBIA — Pollution

POLONIAPHOBIA — Poland (Things Polish)

POLONOPHOBIA — Poles

POLYCRATIPHOBIA — Success

POLYITEROPHOBIA — Multiple Sexual Partners

POLYPHOBIA — Many Things

PORCUPHOBIA — Pigs

PORNOPHOBIA — Pornographic Pictures

PORPHYROPHOBIA — Purple (Colour or Word)

POSSESSIOPHOBIA — Possession (Being Possessed)

POTAMOPHOBIA — Rivers

POTOPHOBIA — Drink

PRIAPISAPHOBIA — Priapism

PRIMATEPHOBIA — Apes

PROCTOPHOBIA — Rectum

PROSOPHOBIA — Progress

PROTESTANTOPHOBIA — Protestantism

PSELLISMOPHOBIA — Stuttering

PSEUDONECROPHOBIA — Death (Pretended Death)

PSEUDOPATHOPHOBIA — Disease (Imagined Disease)

PSEUDOZOOPHOBIA — Fantasy Animals

PSORAPHOBIA — Itching

PSYCHEPHOBIA — Butterflies

PSYCHOPHOBIA — Mind (The Mind)

PSYCHROPHOBIA — Cold (Being Cold)

PTERONOPHOBIA — Feathers

PTSD-PHOBIA — Post-Traumatic Stress Disorder

PUBERTAPHOBIA — Puberty

PUBICANCERPHOBIA — Pubic Lice

PUPAPHOBIA — Puppets

PYGOPHOBIA — Buttocks

PYROPHOBIA — Fire
PYROSIOPHOBIA — Heartburn

QUADRAPHOBIA — Drawn and Quartered (Being Drawn and Quartered)
QUADRATAPHOBIA — Quadratic Equations
QUARTOPHOBIA — Quartets
QUIRITAREPHOBIA — Crying

RABIPHOBIA — Rabies
RADIOPHOBIA — Radiation (Medical Treatments)
RADONOPHOBIA — Radon
RANIDAPHOBIA — Frogs
RECTOPHOBIA — Rectal Disease
REJECTUPHOBIA — Rejection
RETROPHOBIA — Old Things
RETROTEMPOPHOBIA — Time (Travelling Back in Time)
RHABDOPHOBIA — Beaten in Private (Being Beaten in Private)
RHYPOPHOBIA — Uncleanliness
RHYTIPHOBIA — Wrinkles
RITUALISIPHOBIA — Rituals
ROAD RAGE-PHOBIA — Road Rage
RODENTOPHOBIA — Rats
RUINAPHOBIA — Ruins
RUSSOPHOBIA — Russia (Things Russian)

SAD-PHOBIA — Seasonal Affective Disorder
SALIPHOBIA — Salt
SALIROPHOBIA — Salty Body Fluids
SAMHAINOPHOBIA — Halloween
SARMASSOPHOBIA — Touching (Touching People)
SATANOPHOBIA — Satan

SCABIOPHOBIA — Scabies

SCALATORPHOBIA — Escalators

SCATOPHOBIA — Contamination by Faeces

SCELEROPHOBIA — Bad People

SCHIZOPHRENIPHOBIA — Schizophrenia

SCHOOL-PHOBIA — School (Going to School)

SCIOPHOBIA — Shadows

SCOPOPHOBIA — Watching

SCOTOMAPHOBIA — Blind Areas in the Visual Field

SCOTOPHOBIA — Scotland (Things Scottish)

SCRIPTOPHOBIA — Handwriting in Public

SECRETUPHOBIA — Secrets

SEDATEPHOBIA — Silence

SEISMOSOPHOBIA — Earthquakes

SELACHOPHOBIA — Sharks

SELAPHOBIA — Flashing Lights

SEPARAREPHOBIA — Separation

SEPTOPHOBIA — Decaying Matter

SESQUIPEDALOPHOBIA — Words (Long or Unpronounceable)

SIDERODROMOPHOBIA — Trains

SIDEROPHOBIA — Stars

SIDS-PHOBIA — Sudden Infant Death Syndrome

SINISTROPHOBIA — Left-handedness

SINOPHOBIA — China (Things Chinese)

SITICENTRUPHOBIA — Centre Row (Sitting in the Centre of a Row)

SITOPHOBIA — Food

SMYKHEINOPHOBIA — Smoking

SOCERAPHOBIA — Parents-in-law

SOCIALISMOPHOBIA — Socialism

SOCIOPHOBIA — Social Situations

SOMNOPHOBIA — Sleep

SOPHOPHOBIA — Learning

SORICOMORPHAPAPHOBIA — Moles

SOTERIOPHOBIA — Dependence

SOUTH AMEROPHOBIA — South America (Things South American)

SPACEPHOBIA — Space Travel

SPAMOPHOBIA — Computer Spam

SPECTROPHOBIA — Spectres

SPERMATOPHOBIA — Sperm

SPERMOPHOBIA — Germs

SPHEKSOPHOBIA — Wasps

SPORTS-PHOBIA — Sports

STAREOPHOBIA — Standing Still

STASIBASIPHOBIA — Standing Up

STATUOPHOBIA — Statues

STAUROPHOBIA — Crucifixes

STENOPHOBIA — Narrow Places and Things

STIGMATOPHOBIA — Body Modifications

STRICTUPHOBIA — Stress

STROUTHIOPHOBIA — Ostriches

SUAVISIPHOBIA — Sweetness

SUICIDE-PHOBIA — Suicide

SUPERNATURAPHOBIA — Supernatural (The Supernatural)

SUPERSTITIOPHOBIA — Superstitions

SUSPIRAREPHOBIA — Drains

SYMBIOPHOBIA — Intimacy

SYMBOLOPHOBIA — Symbols

SYMMETROPHOBIA — Symmetry

SYMPHOROPHOBIA — Catastrophe

SYNGENESOPHOBIA — Relatives

SYPHILOPHOBIA — Syphilis

TACHOPHOBIA — Speed

TAENIOPHOBIA — Tapeworms

TANGEREPHOBIA — Touching (Touching Objects or Things)

TAOISIOPHOBIA — Taoism

TAPHEPHOBIA — Buried Alive (Being Buried Alive)

TATTOO-PHOBIA — Tattoos

TAUROPHOBIA — Bulls

TAXOPHOBIA — Tidiness

TECHNOPHOBIA — Technology

TELEOPHOBIA — Ceremonies

TELEPHONOPHOBIA — Telephones

TERATOPHOBIA — Deformed Children

TERATROPHOBIA — Monsters

TERROR-PHOBIA — Terrorism

TETANOPHOBIA — Tetanus

TEXTOPHOBIA — Textures (Certain Textures)

THAASOPHOBIA — Sitting Still

THALASSOPHOBIA — Seas

THANATOPHOBIA — Death

THEATROPHOBIA — Theatres

THEOLOGICOPHOBIA — Theology

THEOPHANIAPHOBIA — Jewellery

THEOPHOBIA — Religion

THERMOPHOBIA — Heat

THURAPHOBIA — Doors

TIGRISOPHOBIA — Tigers

TIMOPHOBIA — Status

TITILLAREPHOBIA — Tickled (Being Tickled)

TMJ-PHOBIA — Temporomandibular Joint Disorder

TOCOPHOBIA — Childbirth

TOMOPHOBIA — Surgery

TOPOEXEROPHOBIA — Dry Places

TOPOHYGROPHOBIA — Damp Places

TOPOPHOBIA — Stage (The Stage)

TORTUROPHOBIA — Pain (Another's)

TOXICOPHOBIA — Poison

TRAUMATOPHOBIA — Trauma

TREMOPHOBIA — Trembling

TRICHINOPHOBIA — Trichinosis

TRICHOPATHOPHOBIA — Hair Disease

TRICHOPHOBIA — Hair

TRISKAIDEKAPHOBIA — Thirteen (Number 13)

TROGLOPHOBIA — Caves

TROPOPHOBIA — Moving (Relocation)

TRYPANOPHOBIA — Injections

TRYPOPHOBIA — Holes

TUBERCULOPHOBIA — Tuberculosis

TUBUPHOBIA — Tunnels

TURISTAPHOBIA — Stomach Upset

TUROPHOBIA — Cheese

TV-PHOBIA — Television

TYRANOPHOBIA — Tyrants

UFO-PHOBIA — UFOs

ULCERISIOPHOBIA — Ulcers

ULULAPHOBIA — Owls

UMBILICUPHOBIA — Navel

UNIFORMOPHOBIA — Uniforms

URANOPHOBIA — Heaven

URODELAPHOBIA — Salamanders

UROPHOBIA — Urine

URSUPHOBIA — Bears

URTICARIAPHOBIA — Hives

VACCINOPHOBIA — Vaccinations

VEHEREVAHTOPHOBIA — Weight Differences

VENTRILOQUAPHOBIA — Ventriloquists
VERMIPHOBIA — Vermin
VESPERTILIOPHOBIA — Bats
VESTIPHOBIA — Clothing
VIOLENTIAPHOBIA — Violence
VIRGINITIPHOBIA — Rape (Being Raped While a Virgin)
VITRICOPHOBIA — Stepfathers
VOODOOPHOBIA — Voodoo
VOXIPHOBIA — Voice (Another's)
VUTEUTHINDIONOPHOBIA — Picnics

WALLOONPHOBIA — Walloon (Things Walloon)
WICCAPHOBIA — Witchcraft

X-PHOBIA — X (Letter)
XANTHOPHOBIA — Yellow (Colour or Word)
XENIAPHOBIA — Foreign Doctors
XENOGLOSSOPHOBIA — Foreign Languages
XENOKLEPTOPHOBIA — Foreign Thieves
XENOPHOBIA — Foreigners
XEROPHOBIA — Dryness
XYLINALINAPHOBIA — Cotton
XYLOPHOBIA — Wood
XYROPHOBIA — Razors

YMOPHOBIA — Contrariness (Being Contrary)

ZELOPHOBIA — Jealousy
ZEMMIPHOBIA — Great Mole Rat (The Great Mole Rat)
ZOMBIEPHOBIA — Zombies
ZOONECROPHOBIA — Dead Bodies (Animals)
ZOOPHOBIA — Animals (Domestic)

References

The following works are major sources for this book and drawn upon in virtually all chapters.

A. Beck, J. Emery and R. Greenberg, *Anxiety Disorders and Phobias: A Cognitive Perspective*, Basic Books, New York, 1991.

R. Campbell, *Psychiatric Dictionary* (5th edition), Oxford University Press, London, 1981.

R. Campbell, *Psychiatric Dictionary* (6th edition), Oxford University Press, London, 1989.

R. Campbell, *Psychiatric Dictionary* (7th edition), Oxford University Press, London, 1996.

R. Campbell, *Psychiatric Dictionary* (8th edition), Oxford University Press, London, 2004.

R. Campbell, *Psychiatric Dictionary* (9th edition), Oxford University Press, London, 2009.

G. Davey, *Phobias: A Handbook of Theory, Research and Treatment*, John Wiley & Sons, New York, 2000.

R. Doctor and A. Kahn, *The Encyclopedia of Phobias, Fears, and Anxieties*, Facts on File, New York, 1989.

R. Doctor and A. Kahn, *The Encyclopedia of Phobias, Fears, and Anxieties* (2nd edition), Facts on File, New York, 2000.

R. Doctor, A. Kahn and C. Adamec, *The Encyclopedia of Phobias* (3rd edition), Facts on File, New York, 2008.

L. Hinsie and R. Campbell, *Psychiatric Dictionary* (3rd edition), Oxford University Press, London, 1960.

L. Hinsie and R. Campbell, *Psychiatric Dictionary* (4th edition), Oxford University Press, London, 1970.

L. Hinsie and J. Shatzky, *Psychiatric Dictionary*, Oxford University Press, London, 1940.

L. Hinsie and J. Shatzky, *Psychiatric Dictionary* (2nd edition), Oxford University Press, London, 1953.

D. Hunt, *No More Fears*, Warner Books, New York, 1988.

S. Juan, *The Odd Sex: Mysteries of Our Weird and Wonderful Sex Lives Explained*, HarperCollins, Sydney, 2001.

M. Lader and T. Uhde, *Fast Facts: Anxiety, Panic and Phobias* (2nd edition), Health Press, London, 2006.

M. Maj, H. Akiskal, J. Lopez-Ibor and A. Okasha (Eds.), *Phobias*, John Wiley & Sons, Milton, 2004.

I. Marks, *Fears and Phobias*, Heinemann Medical Books, London, 1969.

I. Marks, *Fears, Phobias, and Rituals: Panic, Anxiety, and Their Disorders*, Oxford University Press, New York, 1987.

J. Melville, *Phobias and Obsessions*, Coward, McCann & Geoghegan, New York, 1977.

R. Waters, *Phobias Revealed and Explained*, Murdoch Books, Sydney, 2003.

CHAPTER 1: INTRODUCTION

1   E. Bourne, *The Anxiety & Phobia Workbook* (4th edition), New Harbinger Publications, Oakland, California, 2005.

2   R. Kessler, W. Chui, O. Demier, K. Merikangas and E. Walters, "Prevalence, severity, and comorbidity of 12-month DSM-IV disorders in the National Comorbidity Survey Replication", *Archives of General Psychiatry*, 2005, vol. 62, no. 6, pp. 617–627; J. Baker, "War on terror", *The Sydney Morning Herald*, 3 November 2005, pp. 1–4.

3   J. Somers, E. Goldner, P. Waraich and L. Hsu, "Prevalence and incidence studies of anxiety disorders: A systematic review of the literature", *Canadian Journal of Psychiatry*, 2006, vol. 51, no. 2, pp. 100–113.

4   L. Lampe, T. Slade, C. Issakidis and G. Andrews, "Social phobia in the Australian National Survey of Mental Health and Well-Being (NSMHWB)", *Psychological Medicine*, 2003, vol. 33, no. 4, pp. 637–646.

5   A. Kleinman, *The Illness Narratives: Suffering, Healing, and the Human Condition*, Basic Books, New York, 1989.

6   L. Kirmayer, "The place of culture in psychiatric nosology: *Taijin kyofusho* and DSM-III-R", *Journal of Nervous Mental Disease*, 1991, vol. 179, no. 1, pp. 19–28.

7   K. Suzuki, N. Takei, M. Kawai, Y. Minabe and N. Mori, "Is *taijin kyofusho* a culture-bound syndrome?", *American Journal of Psychiatry*, 2003, vol. 160, no. 7, p. 1358.

8   K. Hugdahl, *Psychophysiology: The Mind–Body Perspective*, Harvard University Press, Cambridge, Massachusetts, 1996, p. 27.

9   S. Mineka and R. Zinberg, "A contemporary learning theory perspective on the etiology of anxiety disorders: It's not what you thought it was", *American Psychologist*, 2006, vol. 61, no. 1, pp. 10–26.

10 S. Hoffman and M. Otto, *Cognitive Behavioral Therapy for Social Anxiety Disorder*, Routledge, London, 2008, p. 86.

11 G. Davey, *Phobias: A Handbook of Theory, Research and Treatment*, Wiley, New York, 2000, p. 340.

12 Martin Seligman is a professor of psychology at the University of Pennsylvania.

13 M. Seligman, *Biological Boundaries of Learning*, Appleton-Century-Crofts, New York, 1972.

14 R. Peurifoy, *Anxiety, Phobias, & Panic,* Warner Books, New York, 1995.

15 E. Eckert, L. Heston and T. Bouchard, "MZ twins reared apart: Preliminary findings of psychiatric disturbances and traits", *Progress in Clinical and Biological Research*, 1981, vol. 69, part B, pp. 179–188.

16 N. Doidge, *The Brain That Changes Itself,* Penguin Books, New York, 2007; A. Curran, *The Little Book of Big Stuff About the Brain,* The Cromwell Press, Trowbridge, Wiltshire, 2008; J. Allen, *The Lives of the Brain: Human Evolution and the Organ of Mind*, Belknap Press of Harvard University Press, Cambridge, Massachusetts, 2009.

17 L. Hinsie and J. Shatzky, *Psychiatric Dictionary*, Oxford University Press, London, 1940, pp. 218–221.

18 R. Campbell, *Campbell's Psychiatric Dictionary* (9th edition), Oxford University Press, London, 2009, pp. 248–250.

19 American Psychiatric Association, *Diagnostic and Statistical Manual of Mental Disorders*, American Psychiatric Association, Washington, DC, 1952.

20 American Psychiatric Association, *Diagnostic and Statistical Manual of Mental Disorders* (4th edition), American Psychiatric Association, Washington, DC, 2000.

21 E. Stengel, "Classification of mental disorders", *Bulletin of the World Health Organization*, 1959, vol. 21, pp. 601–623.

22 I. Marks, *Fears and Phobias*, Heinemann Medical Books, London, 1969, p. 117.

23 American Psychiatric Association, *Diagnostic and Statistical Manual of Mental Disorders* (3rd edition revised), American Psychiatric Association, Washington, DC, 1987, pp. 240–245.

24 I. Marks, *Fears and Phobias*, Heinemann Medical Books, London, 1969, pp. 76, 108–109, 113, 161.

25 I. Marks, *Fears and Phobias*, Heinemann Medical Books, London, 1969, pp. 70, 75–76.

26 S. Bere, "An atlas of fear", *Popular Science*, January 2008, p. 54.

27 Dr Jitender Sareen and colleagues are from the Department of Psychiatry and Community Health Sciences at the University of Manitoba; J. Sareen, F. Jacobi, B. Cox, S. Belik, I. Clara and M. Stein, "Disability and poor quality of life associated with comorbid anxiety disorders and physical conditions", *Archives of Internal Medicine*, 2006, vol. 166, no. 19, pp. 2109–2116; "Anxiety disorders linked to physical conditions", *Science Daily*, 24 October 2006, p. 1.

28 M. Rutter, J. Tizzard and K. Whitmore, *Education, Health and Behaviour*, Longman's, London, 1968, p. 162.

29 E. Hagman, "A study of fears of children of pre-school age", *Journal of Experimental Education*, 1932, vol. 1, pp. 110–130.

30 E. Becker, M. Rinck, V. Turke, P. Kause, R. Goodwin, S. Neumer and J. Margraf, "Epidemiology of specific phobia subtypes: Findings from the Dresden Mental Health Study", *European Psychiatry*, 2007, vol. 22, no. 2, pp. 69–74.

CHAPTER 2: PHOBIAS STARTING WITH A

1 Cases in this book have been edited for purposes of space and clarity. The age and gender of the person is indicated where it was reported.

2 Many of the celebrity fears and phobias are drawn from internet sources. The information obtained from internet sources should always be

considered with healthy scepticism. "Celebrity Fears and Phobias", http://showbiz.sky.com/celebrity-phobias (retrieved 06–12–2009).

3   T. Carrada-Bravo, "Progressive human viral encephalitis associated with a bat bite", *Neurologia*, 2006, vol. 21, no. 4, pp. 171–175.

4   R. Doctor and A. Kahn, *The Encyclopedia of Phobias, Fears, and Anxieties*, Facts on File, New York, 1989, p. 351.

5   Eremophobia was not included in the list of fears in the first edition of the *Psychiatric Dictionary* in 1940, but was added in the sixth edition in 1989; R. Doctor and A. Kahn, *The Encyclopedia of Phobias, Fears, and Anxieties*, Facts on File, New York, 1989, pp. 28, 206.

6   S. Freud, "Analysis of a phobia in a five-year-old boy (1909)", in S. Freud, *Collected Papers* (Volume 3), Hogarth, London, 1924–1950, pp. 149–287; R. Doctor and A. Kahn, *The Encyclopedia of Phobias, Fears, and Anxieties*, Facts on File, New York, 1989, pp. 32–34; I. Marks, *Fears and Phobias*, Heinemann Medical Books, London, 1969, p. 16.

7   "Celebrity Fears and Phobias", http://showbiz.sky.com/celebrity-phobias (retrieved 06–12–2009).

8   B. Wolf, "Wolf Files: Celebrity Phobias", *ABC News* (New York), http://abcnews.go.com/Entertainment/WolfFiles/story?id=116591&page=1 (retrieved 21–11–2009); "Johnny Depp is Afraid of Clowns: Celebrity Phobias", www.listafterlist.com/DesktopModules/iBelong.LAL.ListRes (retrieved 20–11–2009); "Celebrity Phobias — WhatRumors — The Celebrity Gossip Wiki", www.whatrumors.com/Celebrity_Phobias (retrieved 24–11–2009).

CHAPTER 3: PHOBIAS STARTING WITH B

1   Scelerophobia was not included in the list of fears in the first edition of the *Psychiatric Dictionary* in 1940, but was added in the fourth edition in 1970; R. Campbell, *Psychiatric Dictionary* (8th edition), Oxford University Press, London, 2004, pp. 486; O. James, *They F*** You Up: How to Survive Family Life*, Bloomsbury, London, 2002, p. 221; "Speck", www.unusualphobias.com/speck.html (retrieved 19–02–2006).

2   "Geniusbeauty.com — Celebrity Fears and Phobias Celebrity Phobias",
     http://geniusbeauty.com/celebrity-gossip/celebrity-fears-phobias
     (retrieved 23–11–2009).

3   "Geniusbeauty.com — Celebrity Fears and Phobias Celebrity Phobias",
     http://geniusbeauty.com/celebrity-gossip/celebrity-fears-phobias
     (retrieved 23–11–2009); "Samanda's Fishy Phobia", http://showbiz.
     sky.com/celebrity-phobias (retrieved 06–12–2009); "Balloons", www.
     unusualphobias.com/balloons.html (retrieved 19–02–2006).

4   R. Doctor and A. Kahn, *The Encyclopedia of Phobias, Fears, and Anxieties*,
     Facts on File, New York, 1989, pp. 210, 356.

5   "Celebrity Phobias — WhatRumors — The Celebrity Gossip Wiki",
     www.whatrumors.com/Celebrity_Phobias (retrieved 24–11–2009).

6   Mastigophobia was not included in the list of fears in the first edition of
     the *Psychiatric Dictionary* in 1940, but was added in the sixth edition in
     1989.

7   "Famous People with Animal Phobias", www.bukisa.com/articles/
     195989_famous-people-with animals (retrieved 09–12–2009).

8   Negrophobia was dropped from the list of fears in the eighth edition of the
     Psychiatric Dictionary in 2004, but was reinstated in the ninth edition in 2009.

9   R. Doctor and A. Kahn, *The Encyclopedia of Phobias, Fears, and Anxieties*,
     Facts on File, New York, 1989, pp. 80–81; K. Hellstrom, J. Fellenius and L.
     Ost, "One versus five sessions of applied tension in the treatment of blood
     phobia", *Behaviour Research and Therapy*, 1996, vol. 34, no. 2, pp. 101–102;
     M. Wenner, "Why does blood make some people squeamish but not
     others?", *Popular Science*, March 2008, p. 84.

10   Automysophobia was not included in the list of fears in the first edition of
     the *Psychiatric Dictionary* in 1940, but was added in the eighth edition in
     2004.

11   "Johnny Depp is Afraid of Clowns: Celebrity Phobias", www.listafterlist.
     com/DesktopModules/iBelong.LAL.ListRes (retrieved 20–11–2009).

12   T. Strong, "Eugene Pallette", www.tedstrong.com/eugenepallette.shtml
     (retrieved 28–05–2010).

13   Bibliophobia was not included in the list of fears in the first edition of the
     Psychiatric Dictionary in 1940, but was added in the fourth edition in 1970.

14 Merinthophobia was not included in the list of fears in the first edition of the *Psychiatric Dictionary* in 1940, but was added in the ninth edition in 2009.

15 Gephyrophobia as the fear of bridges was dropped from the list of fears in the sixth edition of the *Psychiatric Dictionary* in 1989 and became fear of "(crossing a) bridge or river"; "PhamousPhobics", www.unusualphobias. com/PhamousPhobics.html (retrieved 08–12–2009); I. Marks, *Fears and Phobias*, Heinemann Medical Books, London, 1969, p. 8.

16 "Celebrity Phobias — WhatRumors — The Celebrity Gossip Wiki", www.whatrumors.com/Celebrity_Phobias (retrieved 24–11–2009).

17 S. Heller, *The Complete Idiot's Guide to Conquering Fear and Anxieties*, Alpha Books, New York, 1999, p. 3.

18 A. Harrington and N. Harrington, "Phobias and Obsessions", http://omg. yahoo.com/news/celebrity-phobias-and-obsessions/253 (retrieved 08–11–2009); "Celebrity Phobias — What They Fear Most", www.popeater. com/2008/10/29/celebrity-phobia-what-they (retrieved 18–11–2009); P. Jones, "I'm a Celebrity … line-up revealed — Blogs — Radio Times", www.radiotimes.com/blogs/469-news-im-a-celebrity-get-me (retrieved 05–12–2009).

19 R. Glover, Richard Glover programme, 702 ABC Radio (Sydney), 17 June 2009.

CHAPTER 4: PHOBIAS STARTING WITH C

1 Carcinomatophobia was not included in the list of fears in the first edition of the *Psychiatric Dictionary* in 1940, but was added in the eighth edition in 2004; P. Hastings, "Remove Phobias, Hypnosis, and NLP", www. realsmart-hypnosis.com/phobias2.html (retrieved 08–12–2009); B. Wolf, "Wolf Files: Celebrity Phobias", *ABC News* (New York), http://abcnews. go.com/Entertainment/WolfFiles/story?id=116591&page=8 (retrieved 21–11–2009).

2 G. Scott, *The History of Corporal Punishment*, T.W. Laurie, London, 1938, p. 147; R. Doctor and A. Kahn, *The Encyclopedia of Phobias, Fears, and Anxieties*, Facts on File, New York, 1989, p. 206.

3   P. Jones, "I'm a Celebrity … line-up revealed — Blogs — Radio Times",
    www.radiotimes.com/blogs/469-news-im-a-celebrity-get-me (retrieved
    05–12–2009).

4   Amaxophobia was dropped from the list of fears in the sixth edition of the
    Psychiatric Dictionary in 1989 and became a less preferred term for fear of
    "vehicles".

5   R. Doctor and A. Kahn, *The Encyclopedia of Phobias, Fears, and Anxieties*,
    Facts on File, New York, 1989, p. 163; I. Duncan, *My Life*, Boni and
    Liveright, New York, 1927; J. Forrester and T. Forrester, *Three Stooges:
    The Triumphs and Tragedies of the Most Popular Comedy Team of All Time*,
    Donaldson Books, Los Angeles, 2002, pp. 151–152; N. Christensen, "A
    view on what scares us", *The Daily Telegraph* (Sydney), 9 August 2010, p. 8;
    C. Scott, "It's Friday the 13th: Do you know where your phobias come
    from?", *The San Francisco Chronicle*, 13 August 2010, p. A8.

6   "Celebrity Fears and Phobias", http://showbiz.sky.com/celebrity-phobias
    (retrieved 06–12–2009); "Driving", www.unusualphobias.com/driving.
    html (retrieved 19–02–2006).

7   The research is being carried out at the School of Psychological Sciences
    under the direction of Professor Nick Tarrier and Dr Caroline Williams;
    "Virtual reality offers solution to driving phobias", *Science Daily*,
    30 November 2009, p. 1.

8   R. Doctor and A. Kahn, *The Encyclopedia of Phobias, Fears, and Anxieties*,
    Facts on File, New York, 1989, p. 94; "Phobias of the Rich and Famous",
    www.associatedcontent.com/article/351722/phobias_of_the_rich_and_
    famous_pg2.html?cat=33 (retrieved 09–12–2009); "Celebrity Phobias",
    www.funtrivia.com.submitquiz.cfm?quiz=114126 (retrieved 18–11–2009);
    "Johnny Depp is Afraid of Clowns: Celebrity Phobias", www.listafterlist.
    com/DesktopModules/iBelong.LAL.ListRes (retrieved 20–11–2009).

9   "Cows", www.unusualphobias.com/cows.html (retrieved 19–02–2006);
    "Celebrity Phobias — WhatRumors — The Celebrity Gossip Wiki",
    www.whatrumors.com/Celebrity_Phobias (retrieved 24–11–2009).

10 P. Jones, "I'm a Celebrity … line-up revealed — Blogs — Radio Times",
    www.radiotimes.com/blogs/469-news-im-a-celebrity-get-me (retrieved
    05–12–2009).

11 "Celebrity Phobias — What They Fear Most", www.popeater.com/
    2008/10/29/celebrity-phobia-what-they (retrieved 18–11–2009).

12 I. Marks, *Fears and Phobias*, Heinemann Medical Books, London, 1969,
    pp. 9–10.

13 "Celebrity Phobias — Jennifer Aniston, 10 Oprah Winfrey", www.
    hollyscoop.com/jennifer-aniston/celebrity-phobia_13 (retrieved
    17–11–2009); "Celebrity Phobias — WhatRumors — The Celebrity
    Gossip Wiki", www.whatrumors.com/Celebrity_Phobias (retrieved
    24–11–2009); "Gum", www.unusualphobias.com/animals.html (retrieved
    19–02–2006).

14 I. Marks, *Fears and Phobias*, Heinemann Medical Books, London,
    1969, p. 9; "Famous People with Animal Phobias", www.bukisa.com/
    articles/195989famous-people-with animals (retrieved 09–12–2009).

15 B. Wolf, "Wolf Files: Celebrity Phobias", *ABC News* (New York),
    http://abcnews.go.com/Entertainment/WolfFiles/story?id=
    116591&page=8 (retrieved 21–11–2009).

16 R. Doctor and A. Kahn, *The Encyclopedia of Phobias, Fears, and Anxieties*,
    Facts on File, New York, 1989, p. 313.

17 "PhamousPhobics", www.unusualphobias.com/PhamousPhobics.html
    (retrieved 12–08–2009); C. April, "Red Carpet Phobia Strikes Famous Singer
    with Anxiety Over Fashion", www.anxietyattackslosangeles.com/2009/11/
    red-carpet-phobia-strikes-famous-singer.html (retrieved 06–08–2010).

18 Coulrophobia was not included in the list of fears in the first edition
    of the *Psychiatric Dictionary* in 1940, but was added in the ninth edition
    in 2009; Professor Paul Salkovskis is clinical director of the Maudsley
    Hospital Centre for Anxiety Disorders and Trauma; R. Glover, Richard
    Glover programme, 702 ABC Radio (Sydney), 17 June 2009; "Celebrity
    Phobias — WhatRumors — The Celebrity Gossip Wiki", www.
    whatrumors.com/Celebrity_ Phobias (retrieved 24–11–2009); B. Wolf,
    "Wolf Files: Celebrity Phobias", *ABC News* (New York), http://abcnews.
    go.com/Entertainment/WolfFiles/story?id=116591&page=4 (retrieved
    21–11–2009); A. Harrington and N. Harrington, "Phobias and
    Obsessions", http://omg.yahoo.com/news/celebrity-phobias-and-
    obsessions/253 (retrieved 18–11–2009); "Celebrity Phobias — What They

Fear Most", www.popeater.com/2008/10/29/celebrity-phobia-what-they (retrieved 18–11–2009); F. Rohrer, "Why are clowns scary?", *BBC News Magazine* (London), 16 January 2008.

19   "Celebrity Phobias — Jennifer Aniston, 4 Scarlett Johansson", www. hollyscoop.com/jennifer-aniston/celebrity-phobia_13 (retrieved 17–11–2009); "Celebrity Phobias — What They Fear Most", www.popeater. com/2008/10/29/celebrity-phobia-what-they (retrieved 18–11–2009).

20   "Johnny Depp is Afraid of Clowns: Celebrity Phobias", www. listafterlist.com/DesktopModules/iBelong.LAL.ListRes (retrieved 20–11–2009); B. Wolf, "Wolf Files: Celebrity Phobias", *ABC News* (New York), http://abcnews.go.com/Entertainment/WolfFiles/story?id= 116591&page=1 (retrieved 21–11–2009).

21   "Celebrities and Their Phobias", www.femalefirst.co.uk/celebrity/ Cheryl+Cole-23101.html (retrieved 27–11–2009).

22   "PhamousPhobics", www.unusualphobias.com/PhamousPhobics.html (retrieved 12–08–2009); B. Wolf, "Wolf Files: Celebrity Phobias", *ABC News* (New York), http://abcnews.go.com/Entertainment/WolfFiles/ story?id=116591&page=8 (retrieved 21–11–2009).

CHAPTER 5: PHOBIAS STARTING WITH D

1   R. Burton, *The Anatomy of Melancholy*, H. Cripps, London, 1621, pp. 143–144; I. Marks, *Fears and Phobias*, Heinemann Medical Books, London, 1969, p. 8; R. Doctor and A. Kahn, *The Encyclopedia of Phobias, Fears, and Anxieties*, Facts on File, New York, 1989, p. 206; "Celebrity Phobias — WhatRumors — The Celebrity Gossip Wiki", www.whatrumors.com/ Celebrity_Phobias (retrieved 24–11–2009); "Celebrity Phobias — Jennifer Aniston, 7 Keanu Reeves", www.hollyscoop.com/jennifer-aniston/ celebrity-phobia_13 (retrieved 17–11–2009); "Johnny Depp is Afraid of Clowns: Celebrity Phobias", www.listafterlist.com/DesktopModules/ iBelong.LAL.ListRes (retrieved 05–11–2009); "Samanda's Fishy Phobia", http://showbiz.sky.com/celebrity-phobias (retrieved 06–12–2009); "Celebrity Fears and Phobias", http://showbiz.sky.com/celebrity-phobias (retrieved 06–12–2009).

2   P. Hastings, "Remove Phobias, Hypnosis, and NLP", www.realsmart-hypnosis.com/phobias2.html (retrieved 08–12–2009); "Top 9 Celebrity Phobias — Woman's Passion", www.womanspassions.com/articles/957. html (retrieved 20–11–2009); "Johnny Depp is Afraid of Clowns: Celebrity Phobias", www.listafterlist.com/DesktopModules/iBelong.LAL.ListRes (retrieved 20–11–2009).

3   "Animals", www.unusualphobias.com/animals.html (retrieved 19–02–2006).

4   Thanatophobia was not included in the list of fears in the first edition of the *Psychiatric Dictionary* in 1940, but was added in the sixth edition in 1989; "Famous Phobia Quotes", www.quotemonk.com/quotes/ famous-p/phobia-quotes.html (retrieved 10–12–2009).

5   "Johnny Depp is Afraid of Clowns: Celebrity Phobias", www.listafterlist. com/DesktopModules/iBelong.LAL.ListRes (retrieved 20–11–2009).

6   "Phobias of the Rich and Famous", www.associatedcontent.com/article/ 351722/phobias_of_the_rich_and_famous_pg2.html?cat=33 (retrieved 12–09–2009); P. Hastings, "Remove Phobias, Hypnosis, and NLP", www.realsmart-hypnosis.com/phobias2.html (retrieved 12–08–2009).

7   R. Doctor and A. Kahn, *The Encyclopedia of Phobias, Fears, and Anxieties*, Facts on File, New York, 1989, p. 206; B. Wolf, "Wolf Files: Celebrity Phobias", *ABC News* (New York), http://abcnews.go.com/Entertainment/ WolfFiles/story?id=116591&page=8 (retrieved 21–11–2009).

8   B. Wolf, "Wolf Files: Celebrity Phobias", *ABC News* (New York), http:// abcnews.go.com/Entertainment/WolfFiles/story?id=116591&page=3 (retrieved 21–11–2009).

9   Illyngophobia was not included in the list of fears in the first edition of the *Psychiatric Dictionary* in 1940, but was added in the ninth edition in 2009.

10   R. Doctor and A. Kahn, *The Encyclopedia of Phobias, Fears, and Anxieties*, Facts on File, New York, 1989, p. 154.

11   R. Ellmann, *James Joyce* (2nd edition), Oxford University Press, New York, 1983, p. 514; J. Forrester and T. Forrester, *Three Stooges: The Triumphs and Tragedies of the Most Popular Comedy Team of All Time*, Donaldson Books, Los Angeles, 2002, pp. 151–152; B. Wolf, "Wolf Files: Celebrity Phobias",

ABC News (New York), http://abcnews.go.com/Entertainment/
WolfFiles/story?id=116591&page=8 (retrieved 21–11–2009).

12   "Celebrity Fears and Phobias", http://showbiz.sky.com/celebrity-phobias
(retrieved 12–06–2009).

13   A. Harrington and N. Harrington, "Phobias and Obsessions", http://
omg.yahoo.com/news/celebrity-phobias-and-obsessions/253 (retrieved
11–08–2009).

14   "Plugs", www.unusualphobias.com/plugs.html (retrieved 19–02–2006).

15   Aquaphobia was not included in the list of fears in the first edition of
the *Psychiatric Dictionary* in 1940, but was added in the eighth edition in
2004; "Celebrity Phobias — WhatRumors — The Celebrity Gossip Wiki",
www.whatrumors.com/Celebrity_Phobias (retrieved 24–11–2009).

16   "Top 9 Celebrity Phobias — Woman's Passion", www.womanspassions.
com/articles/957.html (retrieved 20–11–2009).

CHAPTER 6: PHOBIAS STARTING WITH E

1   B. Wolf, "Wolf Files: Celebrity Phobias", *ABC News* (New York),
http://abcnews.go.com/Entertainment/WolfFiles/story?id=116591&
page=7 (retrieved 21–11–2009).

2   B. Wolf, "Wolf Files: Celebrity Phobias", *ABC News* (New York),
http://abcnews.go.com/Entertainment/WolfFiles/story?id=
116591&page=8 (retrieved 21–11–2009); "Celebrity Phobias —
Wellsphere", http://stanford.wellsphere.com/anxiety-article-
phobia/3 (retrieved 19–11–2009); "Celebrity Phobias — WhatRumors —
The Celebrity Gossip Wiki", www.whatrumors.com/Celebrity_Phobias
(retrieved 24–11–2009).

3   Claustrophobia was not included in the list of fears in the first edition
of the *Psychiatric Dictionary* in 1940, but was added in the eighth edition
in 2004; S. Heller, *The Complete Idiot's Guide to Conquering Fear and
Anxieties*, Alpha Books, New York, 1999, p. 3; B. Wolf, "Wolf Files:
Celebrity Phobias", *ABC News* (New York), http://abcnews.go.com/
Entertainment/WolfFiles/story?id=116591&page=2 (retrieved 21–
11–2009); "Phobias of the Rich and Famous", www.associatedcontent.

com/article/351722/phobias_of_the_rich_and_famous_pg2. html?cat=33 (retrieved 09–12–2009); B. Wolf, "Wolf Files: Celebrity Phobias", *ABC News* (New York), http://abcnews.go.com/ Entertainment/WolfFiles/story?id=116591&page=8 (retrieved 21–11– 2009); "PhamousPhobics", www.unusualphobias.com/PhamousPhobics. html (retrieved 08–12–2009); "Celebrity Phobias! —c2w. com-Play, Create, Win. Trivia, Fun and", http://us.com/quizzes/34086-Celebrity-phobias (retrieved 19–11–2009); "Celebrity Phobias — WhatRumors — The Celebrity Gossip Wiki", www.whatrumors.com/Celebrity_Phobias (retrieved 24–11–2009); P. Hastings, "Remove Phobias, Hypnosis, and NLP", www.realsmart-hypnosis.com/phobias2.html (retrieved 08–12–2009).

4   Erotophobia was not included in the list of fears in the first edition of the *Psychiatric Dictionary* in 1940, but was added in the eighth edition in 2004.

5   "Escalators", www.unusualphobias.com/escalators.html (retrieved 19–02–2006).

6   R. Fulton, "I'm a Celebrity: I'll be showing off my body in the jungle shower, promises Sam Fox", *The Daily Record* (Glasgow), www. dailyrecord.co.uk/showbiz/television-news/2009/11/12 (retrieved 05–12–2009); P. Jones, "I'm a Celebrity … line-up revealed — Blogs — Radio Times", www.radiotimes.com/blogs/469-news-im-a-celebrity-get-me (retrieved 05–12–2009).

CHAPTER 7: PHOBIAS STARTING WITH F

1   Coprophobia was not included in the list of fears in the first edition of the *Psychiatric Dictionary* in 1940, but was added in the eighth edition in 2004.

2   Phobophobia was not included in the list of fears in the first edition of the *Psychiatric Dictionary* in 1940, but was added in the eighth edition in 2004.

3   "Celebrity Phobias", *Cosmopolitan*, www.cosmopolitan.com.au/celebrity_fears_and_phobias.htm (retrieved 27–11–2009).

4   R. Doctor and A. Kahn, *The Encyclopedia of Phobias, Fears, and Anxieties*, Facts on File, New York, 1989, pp. 191, 356.

5 B. Wolf, "Wolf Files: Celebrity Phobias", *ABC News* (New York), http://abcnews.go.com/Entertainment/WolfFiles/story?id=116591&page=6 (retrieved 21–11–2009).

6 "Samanda's Fishy Phobia", http://showbiz.sky.com/celebrity-phobias (retrieved 06–12–2009); "Celebrity Reveal Wacky Phobias", www.exposay.com/celebrities-reveal-wacky-phobias/v/14175/ (retrieved 27–11–2009); "Fish", www.unusualphobias.com/fish.html (retrieved 19–02–2006).

7 "Cracks", www.unusualphobias.com/cracks.html (retrieved 19–02–2006).

8 "Phobias of the Rich and Famous", www.associatedcontent.com/article/351722/phobias_of_the_rich_and_famous_pg2.html?cat=33 (retrieved 09–12–2009).

9 Aviophobia was not included in the list of fears in the first edition of the *Psychiatric Dictionary* in 1940, but was added in the sixth edition in 1989; J. Forrester and T. Forrester, *Three Stooges: The Triumphs and Tragedies of the Most Popular Comedy Team of All Time*, Donaldson Books, Los Angeles, 2002, pp. 151–152; B. Wolf, "Wolf Files: Celebrity Phobias", *ABC News* (New York), http://abcnews.go.com/Entertainment/WolfFiles/story?id=116591&page=1-2 (retrieved 21–11–2009); D. Zagata, "Famous Phobics — Associated Content — associatedcontent.com", www.associatedcontent.com/article/369515/famous_phobias.html (retrieved 12–09–2009); V. McClure, "Phobias of the Rich and Famous", *Cool Quiz!*, www.coolquiz.com/trivia/entertainment/entertainment.asp?ci (retrieved 05–12–2009); "Celebrity Phobias — Jennifer Aniston, 8 Jennifer Aniston, Michael Jackson, Joaquin Phoenix, and Colin Farrell", www.hollyscoop.com/jennifer-aniston/celebrity-phobia_13 (retrieved 17–11–2009); "Celebrity Phobias — What They Fear Most", www.popeater.com/2008/10/29/celebrity-phobia-what-they (retrieved 18–11–2009); "High anxiety", *OK! Magazine*, www.ok.co.uk/body/view/13891/High-anxiety (retrieved 05–12–2009); C. Felsenthal, "Phobias: really nothing to fear", *The Prescott Courier* (Prescott, Arizona), 19 March 1978, p. 5; "Celebrity Phobias", www.funtrivia.com.submitquiz.cfm?quiz=114126 (retrieved

18–11–2009); "Celebrity Phobias — WhatRumors — The Celebrity Gossip Wiki", www.whatrumors.com / Celebrity_Phobias (retrieved 24–11–2009); "Celebrities and Their Phobias", www.femalefirst.co.uk/ celebrity / Cheryl+Cole-23101.html (retrieved 27–11–2009); "Cheryl Cole Reveals Strange Phobia: Cotton Wool", http:// fametastic.co.uk/ active / 20081002 / cheryl-cole-reveal (retrieved 28–11–2009); R. Fulton, "I'm a Celebrity: I'll be showing off my body in the jungle shower, promises Sam Fox", *The Daily Record* (Glasgow), www.dailyrecord. co.uk/ showbiz / television-news / 2009 / 11 / 12 (retrieved 05–12–2009); "Samanda's Fishy Phobia", http:// showbiz.sky.com / celebrity-phobias (retrieved 06–12–2009).

10 C. Walder, J. McCraken, M. Herbert, P. James and N. Brewitt, "Psychological intervention in civilian flying phobias. Evaluation and a three-year follow-up", *British Journal of Psychiatry*, 1987, vol. 151, no. 10, pp. 494–498; I. Marks, *Fears and Phobias*, Heinemann Medical Books, London, 1969, p. 11.

11 Psychologists Drs Samantha Smith of Walter Reed Army Hospital and Barbara O. Rothman of Emory University led the study; "New virtual reality technique helps conquer fear of flying, say researchers", *Science Daily*, 11 August 2000, p. 1.

12 "Cheryl Cole Reveals Strange Phobia: Cotton Wool", http:// fametastic. co.uk/ active / 20081002 / cheryl-cole-reveal (retrieved 28–11–2009).

13 Xenophobia was not included in the list of fears in the first edition of the *Psychiatric Dictionary* in 1940, but was added in the eighth edition in 2004.

14 F. Markey and C. Jersild, "Children's fears, dreams, wishes, daydreams, likes, dislikes, pleasant and unpleasant memories", *Monographs of the Society for Research in Child Development*, 1933, vol. 12.

15 Psychologist Dr Carlos David Navarrete led the experiments; "Xenophobia, for men only", *Science Daily*, 5 February 2009, p. 1.

16 H. Edwards, *The Life of Rossini*, Hurst and Blackett, London, 1869, p. 340; J. Roach, "Friday the 13th phobia rooted in ancient history", *National Geographic News,* http:// news.Nationalgeographic.com/ news / 2004 / 02 / 0212040212friday13.html (retrieved 13–11–2009).

17 A. Leigh, "That girl from Shallotte: Ranidaphobia", http://
thatgirlfromshallotte.blogspot.com/2007/10/ranidaphobia.html
(retrieved 17–01–2008).

CHAPTER 8: PHOBIAS STARTING WITH G

1 "Celebrity Phobias — WhatRumors — The Celebrity Gossip Wiki",
www.whatrumors.com/Celebrity_Phobias (retrieved 24–11–2009).
2 Spermophobia was not included in the list of fears in the first edition
of the *Psychiatric Dictionary* in 1940, but was added in the eighth
edition in 2004; "Celebrity Phobias", www.funtrivia.com.submitquiz.
cfm?quiz=114126 (retrieved 18–11–2009); Editors of *Discover* Magazine,
20 Things You Didn't Know About Everything, HarperCollins, New
York, 2008, p. 142; A. Harrington and N. Harrington, "Phobia and
Obsessions", http://omg.yahoo.com/news/celebrity-phobias-and-
obsessions/253 (retrieved 08–11–2009); "Celebrity Phobias and Obsessions
— justjukie", http://jusjukie.i.ph/blogs/jusjukie/2009/07/18/celebrity-
phobia-a (retrieved 19–11–2009); "Top 9 Celebrity Phobias — Woman's
Passion", www.womanspassions.com/articles/957.html (retrieved
20–11–2009); "Famous People with Phobias — Public Spark", www.
publicspark.com/2008/11/24/famous-people-with-phobias (retrieved
12–09–2009).
3 R. Doctor and A. Kahn, *The Encyclopedia of Phobias, Fears, and Anxieties*,
Facts on File, New York, 1989, p. 181, p. 206.
4 Barophobia was not included in the list of fears in the first edition of
the *Psychiatric Dictionary* in 1940, but was added in the eighth edition in
2004.

CHAPTER 9: PHOBIAS STARTING WITH H

1 "Celebrity Reveal Wacky Phobias", www.exposay.com/celebrities-reveal-
wacky-phobias/v/14175/ (retrieved 27–11–2009).
2 Drs Ronald Doctor, Ada Kahn and Christine Adamec are from the
California State University at Northridge; R. Doctor, A. Kahn and

C. Adamec, *The Encyclopedia of Phobias, Fears, and Anxieties* (3rd edition), Facts on File, New York, 2008, p. 260.

3   F. Corchs, J. Mercante, V. Guendler, D. Vieira, M. Moreira, M. Bernik, E. Zuckerman and M. Peres, "Phobias, other psychiatric comorbidities and chronic migraine", *Arquivos de Neuropsiquiatria*, 2006, vol. 64, no. 4, pp. 950–953.

4   R. Doctor and A. Kahn, *The Encyclopedia of Phobias, Fears, and Anxieties*, Facts on File, New York, 1989, p. 206; "Celebrity Phobias", www. funtrivia.com.submitquiz.cfm?quiz=114126 (retrieved 18–11–2009); C. Adams, "Celebrity Phobias", http://nypost.com/p/pagesix/ celebrity_photos/item_yKo2Dv (retrieved 19–11–2009); "Celebrity Phobias — Nicole Kidman", http://hollyscoop.com/nicole-kidman/ celebrity-phobias_1064 (retrieved 18–11–2009); "Celebrity Phobias — WhatRumors — The Celebrity Gossip Wiki", www.whatrumors.com/ Celebrity_Phobias (retrieved 24–11–2009); R. Fulton, "I'm a Celebrity: I'll be showing off my body in the jungle shower, promises Sam Fox", *The Daily Record* (Glasgow), www.dailyrecord.co.uk/showbiz/ television-news/2009/11/12 (retrieved 05–12–2009); P. Jones, "I'm a Celebrity ... line-up revealed — Blogs — Radio Times", www.radiotimes. com/blogs/469-news-im-a-celebrity-get-me (retrieved 02–12–2009); N. Christensen, "A view on what scares us", *The Daily Telegraph* (Sydney), 9 August 2010, p. 8.

5   "Holes2", www.unusualphobias.com/holes2.html (retrieved 19–02–2006).

6   Equinophobia was not included in the list of fears in the first edition of the *Psychiatric Dictionary* in 1940, but was added in the sixth edition in 1989; "Celebrity Phobias — WhatRumors — The Celebrity Gossip Wiki", www.whatrumors.com/Celebrity_Phobias (retrieved 24–11– 2009); "Famous People with Animal Phobias", www.bukisa.com/ articles/195989_famous-people-with animals (retrieved 09–12–2009).

7   S. Heller, *The Complete Idiot's Guide to Conquering Fear & Anxiety*, Alpha Books, New York, 1999, p. 13.

8   Anthropophobia was not included in the list of fears in the first edition of the *Psychiatric Dictionary* in 1940, but was added in the eighth edition in 2004; M. Van Ostrand, "Celebrity Phobias — Film School Rejects",

www.filmschoolrejects.com/humor/what-scares-the-stars.php (retrieved 21–11–2009).

CHAPTER 10: PHOBIAS STARTING WITH I, J & K

1   J. Hamilton, "Needle phobia: A neglected diagnosis", *Journal of Family Practice*, 1995, vol. 41, no. 2, pp. 169–175; "Celebrity Phobias — WhatRumors — The Celebrity Gossip Wiki", www.whatrumors. com/Celebrity_Phobias (retrieved 24–11–2009); "Celebrity Phobias", *Cosmopolitan*, www.cosmopolitan.com.au/celebrity_fears_and_phobias. htm (retrieved 27–11–2009).

2   "Johnny Depp is Afraid of Clowns: Celebrity Phobias", www. listafterlist. com/DesktopModules/iBelong.LAL.ListRes (retrieved 20–11–2009); R. Fulton, "I'm a Celebrity: I'll be showing off my body in the jungle shower, promises Sam Fox", *The Daily Record* (Glasgow), www. dailyrecord.co.uk/showbiz/television-news/12-11-2009/ (retrieved 05–12–2009); "Celebrity Phobias — WhatRumors — The Celebrity Gossip Wiki", www.whatrumors.com/Celebrity_Phobias (retrieved 24–11–2009); "Famous People with Animal Phobias", www.bukisa.com/ articles/195989 famous-people-with animals (retrieved 09–12–2009); P. Jones, "I'm a Celebrity … line-up revealed — Blogs — Radio Times", www.radiotimes.com/blogs/469-news-im-a-celebrity-get-me (retrieved 05–12–2009).

3   "Jewelry", www.unusualphobias.com/jewelry.html (retrieved 19–02–2006).

4   P. Jones, "I'm a Celebrity … line-up revealed — Blogs — Radio Times", www.radiotimes.com/blogs/469-news-im-a-celebrity-get-me (retrieved 12–05–2009).

CHAPTER 11: PHOBIAS STARTING WITH L

1   P. Jones, "I'm a Celebrity … line-up revealed — Blogs — Radio Times", www.radiotimes.com/blogs/469-news-im-a-celebrity-get-me (retrieved 05–12–2009); "Celebrity Phobias — WhatRumors — The Celebrity Gossip Wiki", www.whatrumors.com/Celebrity_Phobias (retrieved 24–11–2009).

2   Phtheirophobia was not included in the list of fears in the first edition of
     the *Psychiatric Dictionary* in 1940, but was added in the ninth edition in
     2009.

3   L. Proenza, "Challenging fear", Commencement address, The University
     of Akron, Akron, Ohio, 15 August 2009, www.uakron.edu/president/
     speeches_statements/?id=816787 (retrieved 07–07–2010).

CHAPTER 12: PHOBIAS STARTING WITH M

1   "Celebrity Phobias — Jennifer Aniston, 9 Tyra Banks", www.hollyscoop.
     com/jennifer-aniston/celebrity-phobia_13 (retrieved 17–11–2009);
     "Celebrity Phobias — WhatRumors — The Celebrity Gossip Wiki",
     www.whatrumors.com/Celebrity_Phobias (retrieved 24–11–2009).

2   "Samanda's Fishy Phobia", http://showbiz.sky.com/celebrity-phobias
     (retrieved 06–12–2009).

3   Phrenophobia was not included in the list of fears in the first edition of the
     Psychiatric Dictionary in 1940, but was added in the ninth edition in 2009.

4   J. Leavesley, *Mere Mortals*, ABC Books, Sydney, 2004, pp. 208–216.

5   D. McDermott, *Goodson, Mark and Bill Todman*, The Museum of Broadcast
     Communications, Chicago, 10 October 2009; "Famous People with
     Animal Phobias", www.bukisa.com/articles/195989_famous-people-with-
     animal-phobias (retrieved 09–12–2009).

6   "Readmind", www.unusualphobias.com/readmind.html (retrieved
     19–02–2006).

7   "Strange Celebrity Phobias — Popular Culture", http://popular-culture.
     families.com/blog/strange-celebrity-phobias (retrieved 19–11–2009).

8   A. Kendon, "Some functions of gaze-direction in social interaction",
     Unpublished paper, Institute of Experimental Psychology, Oxford
     University, 1965.

9   "Celebrity Phobias — What They Fear Most", www.popeater.com/
     2008/10/29/celebrity-phobia-what-they (retrieved 18–11–2009);
     P. Jones, "I'm a Celebrity … line-up revealed — Blogs — Radio Times",
     www.radiotimes.com/blogs/469-news-im-a-celebrity-get-me (retrieved
     05–12–2009).

10 "Museum", www.unusualphobias.com/museum.html (retrieved 19–02–2006).

CHAPTER 13: PHOBIAS STARTING WITH N & O

1 A. Beyerchen, *Scientists Under Hitler: Politics and the Physics Community in the Third Reich*, Yale University Press, New Haven, 1977.

2 Paralipophobia was not included in the list of fears in the first edition of the *Psychiatric Dictionary* in 1940, but was added in the eighth edition in 2004.

3 R. Wilson, *Prometheus Rising*, New Falcon Publications, Reno, 1983.

4 C. Vallentine, "The innate bases of fear", *Journal of Genetic Psychology*, 1930, vol. 37, pp. 394–419.

5 R. Doctor and A. Kahn, *The Encyclopedia of Phobias, Fears, and Anxieties*, Facts on File, New York, 1989, p. 206; "Top 9 Celebrity Phobias — Woman's Passion", www.womanspassions.com/articles/957.html (retrieved 20–11–2009); "Johnny Depp is Afraid of Clowns: Celebrity Phobias", www.listafterlist.com/DesktopModules/iBelong.LAL.ListRes (retrieved 20–11–2009).

6 "Oddnumbers", www.unusualphobias.com/oddnumbers.html (retrieved 19–02–2006).

7 R. Doctor and A. Kahn, *The Encyclopedia of Phobias, Fears, and Anxieties*, Facts on File, New York, 1989, pp. 292–293.

8 "Ostriches", www.unusualphobias.com/ostriches.html (retrieved 19–02–2006).

9 C. Adams, "Celebrity Phobias", http://nypost.com/p/pagesix/celebrity_photos/item_yKo2Dv (retrieved 19–11–2009).

CHAPTER 14: PHOBIAS STARTING WITH P

1 "Paper", www.unusualphobias.com/paper.html (retrieved 19–02–2006).

2 R. Waters, *Phobias Revealed and Explained*, Murdoch Books, Sydney, 2003, p. 51.

3 J. Leavesley, *Mere Mortals*, ABC Books, Sydney, 2004, pp. 328–336.

4   "Celebrity Phobias — Jennifer Aniston, 1 Orlando Bloom", www. hollyscoop.com/jennifer-aniston/celebrity-phobia_13 (retrieved 17–11–2009); "Celebrity Phobias — WhatRumors — The Celebrity Gossip Wiki", www.whatrumors.com/Celebrity_Phobias (retrieved 24–11–2009).

5   M. Van Ostrand, "Celebrity Phobias — Film School Rejects", www.film schoolrejects.com/tag/celebrity-phobias (retrieved 21–11–2009); "Celebrity Phobias — What They Fear Most", www.popeater. com/2008/10/29/celebrity-phobia-what-they (retrieved 18–11–2009); B. Wolf, "Wolf Files: Celebrity Phobias", *ABC News* (New York), http://abcnews.go.com/Entertainment/WolfFiles/story?id=116591& page=6 (retrieved 21–11–2009).

6   B. Wolf, "Wolf Files: Celebrity Phobias", *ABC News* (New York), http://abcnews.go.com/Entertainment/WolfFiles/story?id=116591& page=8 (retrieved 21–11–2009).

7   I. Marks, *Fears and Phobias*, Heinemann Medical Books, London, 1969, p. 8; C. Scott, "It's Friday the 13th: Do you know where your phobias come from?", *The San Francisco Chronicle*, 13 August 2010, p. A8.

8   O. James, *They F*** You Up: How to Survive Family Life*, Bloomsbury, London, 2002, pp. 221–222.

9   C. Felsenthal, "Phobias: Really nothing to fear", *The Prescott Courier* (Prescott, Arizona), 19 March 1978, p. 5.

10   Agoraphobia was not included in the list of fears in the first edition of the *Psychiatric Dictionary* in 1940, but was added in the sixth edition in 1989; "Agoraphobia", http://en.wikipedia.org/wiki/Agoraphobia (retrieved 17–11–2009); I. Marks, *Fears and Phobias*, Heinemann Medical Books, London, 1969, p. 9; "Famous People with Phobias — Public Spark", www.publicspark.com/2008/11/24/famous-people-with-phobias (retrieved 09–12–2009); E. Weiss, *Agoraphobia in the Light of Ego Psychology*, Grune and Stratton, London, 1964, p. 110; P. Hastings, "Remove Phobias, Hypnosis, and NLP", www.realsmart-hypnosis. com/phobias2.html (retrieved 08–12–2009); B. Wolf, "Wolf Files: Celebrity Phobias", *ABC News* (New York), http://abcnews.go.com/ Entertainment/WolfFiles/story?id=116591&page=8 (retrieved

21–11–2009); "Olivia Hussey", http://en.wikipedia.org/wiki/Olivia_Hussey (retrieved 17–11–2009); C. Adams, "Celebrity Phobias", http://nypost.com/p/pagesix/celebrity_photos/item_yKo2Dv (retrieved 19–11–2009); "Celebrity Phobias — WhatRumors — The Celebrity Gossip Wiki", www.whatrumors.com/Celebrity_Phobias (retrieved 24–11–2009).

11 "Shyness is Everywhere ... Shy/Socially Phobic Celebrities & Everyday People", www.shakeyourshyness.com./shypeople.htm (retrieved 28–11–2009); "Geniusbeauty.com — Celebrity Fears and Phobias Celebrity Phobias", http://geniusbeauty.com/celebrity-gossip/celebrity-fears-phobias (retrieved 23–11–2009).

CHAPTER 15: PHOBIAS STARTING WITH Q & R

1 Lagophobia was not included in the list of fears in the first edition of the *Psychiatric Dictionary* in 1940, but was added in the eighth edition in 2004.

2 "Rainbows", www.unusualphobias.com/rainbows.html (retrieved 19–02–2006).

3 Rodentophobia was not included in the list of fears in the first edition of the *Psychiatric Dictionary* in 1940, but was added in the eighth edition in 2004; P. Jones, "I'm a Celebrity ... line-up revealed — Blogs — Radio Times", www.radiotimes.com/blogs/469-news-im-a-celebrity-get-me (retrieved 05–12–2009).

4 "Top 9 Celebrity Phobias — Woman's Passion", www.womanspassions.com/articles/957.html (retrieved 20–11–2009).

5 Enissophobia was not included in the list of fears in the first edition of the *Psychiatric Dictionary* in 1940, but was added in the ninth edition in 2009.

6 "Celebrity Phobias — WhatRumors — The Celebrity Gossip Wiki", www.whatrumors.com/Celebrity_Phobias (retrieved 24–11–2009); "Geniusbeauty.com — Celebrity Fears and Phobias Celebrity Phobias", http://geniusbeauty.com/celebrity-gossip/ celebrity-fears-phobias (retrieved 23–11–2009).

7 Catagelophobia was not included in the list of fears in the first edition of

the *Psychiatric Dictionary* in 1940, but was added in the sixth edition in 1989.

8   R. Doctor and A. Kahn, *The Encyclopedia of Phobias, Fears, and Anxieties*, Facts on File, New York, 1989, p. 313.

CHAPTER 16: PHOBIAS STARTING WITH S

1   School-phobia and Scholionophobia were not included in the list of fears in the first edition of the *Psychiatric Dictionary* in 1940, but were added in the eighth edition in 2004.

2   Hellenologophobia was not included in the list of fears in the first edition of the *Psychiatric Dictionary* in 1940, but was added in the fourth edition in 1970.

3   "Celebrity Phobias — What They Fear Most", www.popeater.com/2008/ 10/29/celebrity-phobia-what-they (retrieved 18–11–2009); "Celebrity Phobias — WhatRumors — The Celebrity Gossip Wiki", www. whatrumors.com/Celebrity_Phobias (retrieved 24–11–2009); "Coral", www.unusualphobias.com/coral.html (retrieved 19–02–2006); "Seacreatures", www.unusualphobias.com/seacreatures.html (retrieved 19–02–2006).

4   Homilophobia was dropped from the list of fears in the third edition of the *Psychiatric Dictionary* in 1960.

5   "Celebrity Phobias — What They Fear Most", www.popeater.com/ 2008/10/29/celebrity-phobia-what-they (retrieved 18–11–2009); B. Wolf, "Wolf Files: Celebrity Phobias", *ABC News* (New York), http://abcnews.go.com/Entertainment/WolfFiles/story?id=116591& page=6 (retrieved 21–11–2009); "Celebrity Phobias — WhatRumors — The Celebrity Gossip Wiki", www.whatrumors.com/Celebrity_Phobias (retrieved 24–11–2009); "Samanda's Fishy Phobia", http://showbiz. sky.com/celebrity-phobias (retrieved 06–12–2009).

6   P. Royle, "Crabs", *Philosophy Now*, May–June 2008, p. 17; "Lobsters", www.unusualphobias.com/lobsters.html (retrieved 19–02–2006).

7   C. Scott, "It's Friday the 13th: Do you know where your phobias come from?", *The San Francisco Chronicle*, 13 August 2010, p. A8.

8   "Shrinking", http://www.unusualphobias.com/shrinking.html (retrieved
    19–02–2006).

9   B. Wolf, "Wolf Files: Celebrity Phobias", *ABC News* (New York),
    http://abcnews.go.com/Entertainment/WolfFiles/story?id=116591&
    page=7 (retrieved 21–11–2009).

10 "Celebrity Phobias", www.funtrivia.com.submitquiz.cfm?quiz=114126
    (retrieved 18–11–2009); C. Felsenthal, "Phobias: Really nothing to fear",
    The Prescott Courier (Prescott, Arizona), 19 March 1978, p. 5; "Celebrity
    Phobias — Jennifer Aniston, 3 Justin Timberlake", www.hollyscoop.
    com/jennifer-aniston/celebrity-phobia_13 (retrieved 17–11–2009);
    "Celebrity Phobias — WhatRumors — The Celebrity Gossip Wiki",
    www.whatrumors.com/Celebrity_Phobias (retrieved 24–11–2009);
    P. Hastings, "Remove Phobias, Hypnosis, and NLP", www.realsmart-
    hypnosis.com/phobias2.html (retrieved 08–12–2009); R. Fulton, "I'm a
    Celebrity: I'll be showing off my body in the jungle shower, promises
    Sam Fox", *The Daily Record* (Glasgow), www.dailyrecord.co.uk/showbiz/
    television-news/2009/11/12 (retrieved 05–12–2009); P. Jones, "I'm a
    Celebrity … line-up revealed — Blogs — Radio Times", www.radiotimes.
    com/blogs/469-news-im-a-celebrity-get-me (retrieved 05–12–2009);
    N. Christensen, "A view on what scares us", *The Daily Telegraph* (Sydney),
    9 August 2010, p. 8.

11 H. Jones and M. Jones, "Motivation and emotion: Fear of snakes",
    Childhood Education, 1928, vol. 5, pp. 136–143; G. Morris and D. Morris,
    Men and Snakes, Hutchinson, London, 1965, pp. 200–215.

12 Psychologist Dr Helena led the study; "Unlocking the psychology of
    snake and spider phobias", *Science Daily*, 24 March 2008, p. 1; H. Purkis
    and O. Lipp, "Automatic attention does not equal automatic fear:
    Preferential attention without implicit valence", *Emotion*, 2007, vol. 7,
    no. 2, pp. 314–323.

13 "Shyness is Everywhere … Shy/Socially Phobic Celebrities & Everyday
    People", www.shakeyourshyness.com./shypeople.htm (retrieved 28–
    11–2009); "Social Phobia Anxiety Disorder — Shyness & Social Anxiety
    Treatment Australia", www.socialanxietyassist.com.au/social_ shtml
    (retrieved 11–12–2009); C. April, "Red Carpet Phobia Strikes Famous

Singer with Anxiety Over Fashion", www.anxietyattackslosangeles. com/2009/11/red-carpet-phobia-strikes-famous-singer.html (retrieved 06–08–2010).

14 Researchers involved in the study were neurophysiologist Dr Pradeep Nathan from the Centre for Brain and Behaviour and the Department of Physiology at Monash University, Drs Luan Phan and Danield Fitzgerald at the University of Chicago, and Dr Manuel Tancer at Wayne State University in Detroit; "Studying brain activity could aid diagnosis of social phobia", *Science Daily*, 19 January 2006, p. 1.

15 Dr Van der Wee is from the Department of Psychiatry and the Leiden Institute for Brain and Cognition at the Leiden University Medical Center; "Are anxiety disorders all in the mind?", *Science Daily*, 12 May 2008, p. 1.

16 Neuroscientist Dr Predrag Petrovic from the Department of Clinical Neuroscience at the Karolinska Institutet led the study; "Hormone oxytocin may inhibit social phobia", *Science Daily*, 23 July 2008, p. 1.

17 Neuropsychologist Dr Karina Blair led the study; "Individuals with social phobia see themselves differently", *Science Daily*, 7 October 2008, p. 1.

18 Phonophobia was not included in the list of fears in the first edition of the *Psychiatric Dictionary* in 1940, but was added in the eighth edition in 2004; B. Wolf, "Wolf Files: Celebrity Phobias", *ABC News* (New York), http://abcnews.go.com/Entertainment/WolfFiles/story?id=116591&page=5 (retrieved 21–11–2009).

19 "Celebrity Phobias — WhatRumors — The Celebrity Gossip Wiki", www.whatrumors.com/Celebrity_Phobias (retrieved 24–11–2009).

20 Tachophobia was not included in the list of fears in the first edition of the *Psychiatric Dictionary* in 1940, but was added in the eighth edition in 2004.

21 A. Ohman and S. Mineka, "Fears, phobias, and preparedness: Toward an evolved module of fear and fear learning", *Psychological Review*, 2001, vol. 108, no. 3, pp. 483–522; C. Scott, "It's Friday the 13th: Do you know where your phobias come from?", *The San Francisco Chronicle*, 13 August 2010, p. A8; L. Ost, "One-session group treatment of spider phobia", *Behaviour Research and Therapy*, 1996, vol. 34, no. 9, pp. 707–715; "Celebrity Phobias — What They Fear Most", www. popeater.com/2008/10/29/celebrity-phobia-what-they (retrieved

18–11–2009); R. Doctor and A. Kahn, *The Encyclopedia of Phobias, Fears, and Anxieties*, Facts on File, New York, 1989, p. 382; "Celebrity Phobias — WhatRumors — The Celebrity Gossip Wiki", www.whatrumors. com/Celebrity_Phobias (retrieved 24–11–2009); P. Hastings, "Remove Phobias, Hypnosis, and NLP", www.realsmart-hypnosis.com/phobias2. html (retrieved 08–12–2009); R. Fulton, "I'm a Celebrity: I'll be showing off my body in the jungle shower, promises Sam Fox", *The Daily Record* (Glasgow), www.dailyrecord.co.uk/showbiz/television-news/2009/11/12 (retrieved 05–12–2009); P. Jones, "I'm a Celebrity … line-up revealed — Blogs — Radio Times", www.radiotimes. com/blogs/469-news-im-a-celebrity-get-me (retrieved 05–12–2009); N. Christensen, "A view on what scares us", *The Daily Telegraph* (Sydney), 9 August 2010, p. 8.

22 Drs Jones and Menzies are from the School of Behavioural and Community Health Sciences at the University of Sydney; M. Jones and R. Menzies, "Danger expectancies, self-efficacy and insight in spider phobia", *Behaviour Research and Therapy*, 2000, vol. 38, no. 6, pp. 585–600.

23 Drs Hunter Hoffman, Albert Carlin and Thomas Furness of the Human Interface Technology Laboratory at the University of Washington, along with Drs Azucena Garcia-Palacios and Cristina Botella-Arbona of Universidad Jaume I in Spain, were involved in the study; "Touch doubles the power of virtual reality therapy for spider phobia", *Science Daily*, 31 October 2003, p. 1.

24 R. Burton, *The Anatomy of Melancholy*, H. Cripps, London, 1621, pp. 143–144; "PhamousPhobics", www.unusualphobias.com/PhamousPhobics. html (retrieved 08–12–2009); S. Heller, *The Complete Idiot's Guide to Conquering Fear and Anxieties*, Alpha Books, New York, 1999, p. 182; I. Marks, *Fears and Phobias*, Heinemann Medical Books, London, 1969, p. 8; "Celebrity Phobias", *Cosmopolitan*, www.cosmopolitan.com.au/ celebrity_fears_and_phobias.htm (retrieved 27–11–2009).

25 Polycratiphobia was not included in the list of fears in the first edition of the *Psychiatric Dictionary* in 1940, but was added in the sixth edition in 1989.

26 B. Wolf, "Wolf Files: Celebrity Phobias", *ABC News* (New York), http://abcnews.go.com/Entertainment/WolfFiles/story?id=116591& page=6 (retrieved 21–11–2009).

CHAPTER 17: PHOBIAS STARTING WITH T

1   "Oneindia.in — Print", www.greynium.com/mail-print/print.php (retrieved 19–11–2009); "Celebrity Phobias — WhatRumors — The Celebrity Gossip Wiki", www.whatrumors.com/Celebrity_Phobias (retrieved 24–11–2009).

2   "Top 9 Celebrity Phobias — Woman's Passion", www.womanspassions. com/articles/957.html (retrieved 20–11–2009).

3   Triskaidekaphobia was not included in the list of fears in the first edition of the *Psychiatric Dictionary* in 1940, but was added in the sixth edition in 1989; Ripley's Believe It or Not!, *Beyond Belief*, Miles Kelly Publishing, Orlando, Florida, 2006, p. 35; V. McClure, "Phobias of the Rich and Famous", *Cool Quiz!*, www.coolquiz.com/trivia/entertainment/ entertainment/.asp?ci (retrieved 05–12–2009).

4   Bathmophobia was not included in the list of fears in the first edition of the *Psychiatric Dictionary* in 1940, but was added in the eighth edition in 2004.

5   A. Harrington and N. Harrington, "Phobias and Obsessions", http:// omg.yahoo.com/news/celebrity-phobias-and-obsessions/253 (retrieved 08–11–2009); R. Ellmann, *James Joyce* (2nd edition), Oxford University Press, New York, 1983, p. 514.

6   N. Botham, *The Best Book of Useless Information Ever*, John Blake, London, 2005, p. 143; "Celebrity Phobias — WhatRumors — The Celebrity Gossip Wiki", www.whatrumors.com/Celebrity_Phobias (retrieved 24–11–2009).

7   "Famous People with Phobias — Public Spark", www.publicspark. com/2008/11/24/famous-people-with-phobias (retrieved 09–12–2009); P. Hastings, "Remove Phobias, Hypnosis, and NLP", www. realsmart-hypnosis.com/phobias2.html (retrieved 08–12–2009); "10 Famous People and Their Phobias", www.toptenz.net/10-famous-people-and-their-phobias.php (retrieved 08–12–2009).

8 "Famous People with Phobias — Public Spark", www.publicspark. com/2008/11/24/famous-people-with-phobias (retrieved 09–12–2009); "Parkingramps", www.unusualphobias.com/parkingramps.html (retrieved 19–02–2006); "Highwaysystem", www.unusualphobias.com/ highwaysystem.html (retrieved 19–02–2006).

9 A. Harrington and N. Harrington, "Phobias and Obsessions", http:// omg.yahoo.com/news/celebrity-phobias-and-obsessions/253 (retrieved 08–11–2009); "Celebrity Phobias — WhatRumors — The Celebrity Gossip Wiki", www.whatrumors.com/Celebrity_Phobias (retrieved 24–11–2009).

10 C. Lockard, "Summer school 09 chelonaphobia?", www.sheldon.k12. mo.us/vnews/display.v/ (retrieved 15–08–2009).

CHAPTER 18: PHOBIAS STARTING WITH U & V

1 O. James, *They F*** You Up: How to Survive Family Life*, Bloomsbury, London, 2002, p. 222; A. Harrington and N. Harrington, "Phobias and Obsessions", http://omg.yahoo.com/news/celebrity-phobias-and-obsessions/253 (retrieved 08–11–2009); "Geniusbeauty.com — Celebrity Fears and Phobias Celebrity Phobias", http://geniusbeauty.com/ celebrity-gossip/celebrity-fears-phobias (retrieved 23–11–2009).

CHAPTER 19: PHOBIAS STARTING WITH W, X, Y & Z

1 Dr Margaret Mary Wilson is a geriatrics specialist at the School of Medicine at Saint Louis University; M. Wilson, D. Miller, E. Andresen, T. Malmstrom, J. Miller and F. Wolinsky, "Fear of falling and related activity restrictions among middle-aged African Americans", *Journals of Gerontology, Series A, Biological Sciences and Medical Sciences*, 2005, vol. 60, no. 3, pp. 355–360; "Fear of falling: It's not only grandpa's phobia", *Science Daily*, 10 May 2005, p. 1.

2 "Phobias of the Rich and Famous", www.associatedcontent.com/article/ 351722/phobias_of_the_rich_and_famous_pg2.html?cat=33 (retrieved 09–12–2009); A. Miller, *For Your Own Good: Hidden Cruelty in Child-Rearing and the Roots of Violence* (2nd edition), Farrar, Strauss, Giroux, New

York, 1984, p. 143; "Curtain", www.unusualphobias.com/curtain.html (retrieved 19–02–2006).

3   P. Hastings, "Remove Phobias, Hypnosis, and NLP", www.realsmart-hypnosis.com/phobias2.html (retrieved 08–12–2009).

4   "Phobias of the Rich and Famous", www.associatedcontent.com/article/351722/phobias_of_the_rich_and_famous_pg2.html?cat=33 (retrieved 09–12–2009); J. Forrester and T. Forrester, *Three Stooges: The Triumphs and Tragedies of the Most Popular Comedy Team of All Time*, Donaldson Books, Los Angeles, 2002, pp. 151–152; P. Jones, "I'm a Celebrity ... line-up revealed — Blogs — Radio Times", www.radiotimes.com/blogs/469-news-im-a-celebrity-get-me (retrieved 05–12–2009); P. Hastings, "Remove Phobias, Hypnosis, and NLP", www.realsmart-hypnosis.com/phobias2.html (retrieved 08–12–2009).

5   "Celebrity Reveal Wacky Phobias", www.exposay.com/celebrities-reveal-wacky-phobias/v/14175/ (retrieved 27–11–2009); "Waterfalls", www.unusualphobias.com/waterfalls.html (retrieved 19–02–2006).

6   R. Kleinknecht, R. Thorndike and M. Walls, "Factorial dimensions and correlates of blood, injury, injection and related medical fears: Cross validation of the medical fear survey", *Behaviour Research and Therapy*, 1996, vol. 34, no. 4, pp. 323–331.

7   "Raccoons", www.unusualphobias.com/speck.html (retrieved 19–02–2006); "Ferrets", www.unusualphobias.com/ferrets.html (retrieved 19–02–2006).

8   "Blowingclothes", www.unusualphobias.com/blowingclothes.html (retrieved 19–02–2006).

9   I. Marks, *Fears and Phobias*, Heinemann Medical Books, London, 1969, pp. 7–8.

10 S. Juan, *The Odd Brain: Mysteries of Our Weird and Wonderful Brains Explained*, HarperCollins, Sydney, 1998, pp. 38–44.

11 Logophobia was not included in the list of fears in the first edition of the *Psychiatric Dictionary* in 1940, but was added in the eighth edition in 2004.

12 R. Glover, Richard Glover programme, 702 ABC Radio (Sydney), 17 June 2009; "Worms", www.unusualphobias.com/worms.html (retrieved 19–02–2006).

13 R. Descartes, *Discourse on Method and Meditations* (1637), The Liberal Arts Press, New York, 1960.

CHAPTER 20: OUR EVOLUTION IN PHOBIA UNDERSTANDING

1   I. Marks, *Fears and Phobias*, Heinemann Medical Books, London, 1969, pp. 7–12, 70, 94.
2   J. Shine, "Some Phobias in the Past", *International Quantum Healing*, www.internationalquantumhealing.com (retrieved 09–12–2009).
3   R. Descartes, *The Passions of the Soule*, Martin and Ridley, London, 1650, pp. 107–108.
4   J. Locke, *The Philosophical Works of John Locke*, G. Bell, London, 1913, p. 212.
5   C. Westphal, *"Die agoraphobie: eine neuropathische erscheinung"*, *Archiv fur Psychiatrie und Nervenkrankheiten*, 1871–1872, vol. 3, pp. 138–171, 219–221.
6   C. Darwin, *On the Expression of Emotions in Man and Animals*, John Murray, London, 1872.
7   R. Doctor, A. Kahn and C. Adamec, *The Encyclopedia of Phobias* (3rd edition), Facts on File, New York, 2008, pp. xiv–xv.
8   H. Maudsley, *The Pathology of Mind*, Macmillan, London, 1879, pp. 409–411.
9   G. Hall, "A study of fears", *American Journal of Psychology*, 1897, vol. 8, pp. 147–249.
10 S. Freud, "The justification for detaching from neurasthenia a particular syndrome: The anxiety neurosis (1894)", in S. Freud, *Collected Papers* (Volume 1), Hogarth, London, 1924–1950, pp. 78–106.
11 E. Kraepelin, *Psychologische Arbeiten*, W. Engelmann, Leipzig, 1895–1921.
12 J. Watson and R. Rayner, "Conditioned emotional reactions", *Journal of Experimental Psychology*, 1920, vol. 3, pp. 1–14; H. English, "Three cases of the 'conditioned fear response'", *Journal of Abnormal Social Psychology*, 1929, vol. 34, pp. 221–225.
13 B. Lewin, "Phobic symptoms and dream interpretation", *Psychoanalytic Quarterly*, 1952, vol. 21, pp. 295–321.

14 S. Agras, D. Sylvester and D. Oliveau, "The epidemiology of
    common fears and phobias", *Comprehensive Psychiatry*, 1969, vol. 10,
    pp. 151–156.

15 H. Adams and P. Sutker, *Comprehensive Handbook of Psychopathology*,
    Plenum Press, New York, 1984, p. vii.

16 T. Straube, H. Mentzel, M. Glauer and W. Miltner, "Brain activation
    to phobia-related words in phobic subjects", *Neuroscience Letters*, 2004,
    vol. 372, no. 3, pp. 204–208.

17 O. Mowrer, *Leaves From Many Seasons: Selected Papers*, Praeger, New York,
    1983.

18 Dr Jeffrey Lohr is a psychologist at the University of Arkansas in
    Fayetteville; "University of Arkansas researchers tease out the role of
    disgust in phobias", *Science Daily*, 27 November 2002, p. 1.

19 Dr Christine Albert is from the Division of Preventive Medicine at
    Harvard Medical School; C. Albert, C. Chae, K. Rexrode, J. Manson
    and I. Kawachi, "Phobic anxiety and risk of coronary heart disease and
    sudden cardiac death among women", *Circulation*, 2005, vol. 111, no. 4,
    pp. 480–487; "Phobic anxiety increases heart disease death risk among
    women", *Science Daily*, 9 February 2005, p. 1.

20 Dr Li-Huei Tsai is a neuroscientist at the Department of Brain and
    Cognitive Sciences at MIT; "Mechanism behind fear discovered", *Science
    Daily*, 22 July 2007, p. 1.

21 Dr Franziska Geiser is from the Clinic and Policlinic for Psychosomatic
    Medicine and Psychotherapy and Dr Ursula Harbrecht is from the
    Institute of Experimental Haematology and Transfusion Medicine at the
    University of Bonn; "Anxiety linked to blood clots: Fear that freezes the
    blood in your veins", *Science Daily*, 28 March 2008, p. 1.

22 A. Ohman and S. Mineka, "Fears, phobias, and preparedness: Toward
    an evolved module of fear and fear learning", *Psychological Review*, 2001,
    vol. 108, no. 3, pp. 483–522; C. Scott, "It's Friday the 13th: Do you know
    where your phobias come from?", *The San Francisco Chronicle*, 13 August
    2010, p. A8.

CHAPTER 21: TREATMENT

1   C. Antoniades, "Tips for treating your phobias", *The Washington Post*, 10 August 2006, p. N04; C. Antoniades, "Fear factors", *The Washington Post*, 10 August 2006, p. N01; J. Ross and R. Carter, *Triumph Over Fear: A Book of Help and Hope for People with Anxiety, Panic Attacks and Phobias*, Bantam Books, New York, 1995; H. Saul, *Phobias: Fighting the Fear*, HarperCollins, London, 2001.

2   J. Wolpe, *Psychotherapy by Reciprocal Inhibition*, Stanford University Press, Palo Alto, 1958; F. Shapiro, *Eye Movement Desensitization and Reprocessing: Basic Principles, Protocols, and Procedures*, Guildford Press, New York, 2001; R. Doctor, A. Kahn and C. Adamec, *The Encyclopedia of Phobias* (3rd edition), Facts on File, New York, 2008, p. xvii; I. Marks, *Fears and Phobias*, Heinemann Medical Books, London, 1969, p. 88.

3   Y. Choy, A. Fyer and J. Lipsitz, "Treatment of specific phobia in adults", *Clinical Psychology Review*, 2007, vol. 27, no. 3, pp. 266–286.

4   Dr Mark Barad is from the Neuropsychiatric Institute of UCLA; "Scientists find more efficient way to 'unlearn' fear", *Science Daily*, 6 October 2003, p. 1.

5   "Biology of fear", *Science Daily*, 5 April 2004, p. 1.

6   J. Baker, "When fear takes over", *The Sydney Morning Herald*, 28 May 2009, pp. 1–2.

7   R. Rapee, M. Abbott, A. Baillie and J. Gaston, "Treatment of social phobia through pure self-help and therapist-augmented self-help", *British Journal of Psychology*, 2007, vol. 191, pp. 246–252; "Self-help treatment for social anxiety can ease burden", *Science Daily*, 15 October 2007, p. 1.

8   Dr Elizabeth Phelps and colleagues are from the Department of Psychology and the Center for Neural Science at New York University; D. Schiller, M. Monfils, C. Raio, D. Johnson, J. LeDoux and E. Phelps, "Preventing the return of fear in humans using reconsolidation update mechanisms", *Nature*, 2010, vol. 463, no. 7277, pp. 49–53; "Noninvasive technique to rewrite fear memories developed", *Science Daily*, 10 December 2009, p. 1.

9   M. Yoshida and R. Hirano, "Effects of local anesthesia of the cerebellum
     on classical fear conditioning in goldfish", *Behavioral and Brain Functions*,
     2010, vol. 6, p. 20; "Fearless fish forget their phobias", *Science Daily*,
     23 March 2010, p. 1.

CHAPTER 22: CHILDHOOD PHOBIAS

1   R. Fantz, "Pattern vision in newborn infants", *Science*, 1963, vol. 140 (3564),
     pp. 296–297.
2   S. Rachman and C. Costello, "The aetiology and treatment of
     children's phobias: A review", *American Journal of Psychiatry*, 1961,
     vol. 118, no. 8, pp. 97–105; N. King, G. Eleonora and T. Ollendick,
     "The etiology of childhood dog phobia", *Behaviour Research and Therapy*,
     1997, vol. 35, no. 1, p. 77; N. King, G. Eleonora and T. Ollendick,
     "Etiology of childhood phobias: Current status of Rachman's three
     pathways theory", *Behaviour Research and Therapy*, 1998, vol. 36, no. 3,
     pp. 297–309.
3   A. Bandura and T. Rosenthal, "Vicarious classical conditioning as a
     function of arousal level", *Journal of Personality and Social Psychology*, 1966,
     vol. 3, pp. 54–62.
4   L. Cooke, C. Haworth and J. Wardle, "Genetic and environmental
     influences on children's food neophobia", *American Journal of Clinical
     Nutrition*, 2007, vol. 86, no. 2, pp. 428–433.
5   M. Jones, "A laboratory study of fear: The case of Peter", *Journal of
     Pediatric Seminars*, 1924, vol. 31, pp. 308–315.
6   "Half of group free of phobia after a single treatment", *Science Daily*,
     31 March 2009, p. 1.
7   Research Unit on Pediatric Psychopharmacology Anxiety Study Group,
     National Institute of Mental Health, "Fluvoxamine for the treatment of
     anxiety disorders in children and adolescents", *The New England Journal
     of Medicine*, 2001, vol. 344, no. 17, pp. 1279–1285; "Medication effective
     in treating anxiety disorders in children and adolescents", *Science Daily*,
     4 May 2001, p. 1.

8   C. Last and C. Strauss, "School refusal in anxiety-disordered children and adolescents", *Journal of the American Academy of Child and Adolescent Psychiatry*, 1990, vol. 29, no. 1, pp. 31–35.

9   H. Merckelbach, P. Muris and E. Schouten, "Pathways to fear in spider phobic children", *Behaviour Research and Therapy*, 1996, vol. 34, nos. 11–12, pp. 935–938; P. Muris, H. Merckelbach and R. Collaris, "Common childhood fears and their origins", *Behaviour Research and Therapy*, 1997, vol. 35, no. 10, pp. 929–937.

Acknowledgements

Besides the author, there are many individuals who work together to produce a book. At HarperCollins Australia in Sydney these include Michael Moynahan, the CEO, Shona Martyn, the publishing director, Julian Gray, my publisher, Beth Conway, the international rights associate, Melanie Peake, my website manager, Caitlin Beyer in reception and everyone in production. Thanks to Josh Durham, the cover designer. Thanks to Kate Burnitt for doing such a wonderful job of editing a rather difficult manuscript. Thanks to Sarina Rowell and Emma Schwarcz for proofreading. Thanks to those in the publicity team, led by Christine Farmer: Nicola Howcroft, Jane Finemore, Laura Benson, Jace Armstrong, Eliza Segal, Kelly Fagan and Grace McBride. Finally, major thanks should go to the HarperCollins Australia sales reps for their many years of going out into the bookshop world and urging booksellers to once again, "Take a look at another Dr Stephen Juan title": Steve Howard, Jodi Collas, Denis Phillips, Michael Hanley, Maurice Baker, Jacqui Furlong, Brigita Rakas, Nigel Page, Maria Tsiakopoulos, Erin Dunk, John Williams, Toni Halley, Anthony Little, Graeme Sinclair, Theresa Anns, Ian Vanderfeen, Susie Jarrett, Kathleen Hendry and their manager, Sue Brodie.

Thanks are owed to the researchers, authors and publishers of the many research findings mentioned in this book. Among these is Professor Isaac Marks of the University of London. His pioneering work in phobias and fears has been the benchmark in this field. Hopefully, he will not be too annoyed that an anthropologist has somewhat modified his classification system of phobias formulated some 40 years ago.

Thanks are owed to the staff at the University of Sydney libraries, the National Library of Australia in Canberra, the US Library of Congress, the US National Library of Medicine and the US National Institutes of Health in Washington, DC.

Thanks also to the book publishers around the world who have published foreign language editions of my various books.

Thanks to the radio and TV station hosts and producers who continually invite me on to their programmes.

Thanks to the individuals who supplied descriptions of their phobias. Obviously I cannot name them but I am appreciative that they shared their stories.

Thanks to my friends and colleagues who shared ideas with me about this book and ideas related to it, especially Michele Knight, Ian Stevens, Dr Nina Burridge, Dr Richard Walker, Dr Ray Younis and Sharon Dean.

Stephen Juan, Ph.D.

About the Author

Dr Stephen Juan is the author of 13 books, including *The Odd Body* (1995), *The Odd Brain* (1998), *The Odd Body 2* (2000), *The Odd Sex* (2001), *The Odd Body 3* (2007) and *Can Kissing Make You Live Longer?* (2010), all published by HarperCollins Australia.

Scientist, educator and journalist, Dr Juan is an anthropologist by training and one of the world's best communicators of research. His various books have been translated into 27 languages. He has served as a magazine editor and a newspaper columnist for papers such as *The Sydney Morning Herald*, *The Sun-Herald* (Sydney), *The National Post* (Toronto), *The New York Daily News* and *The Register* (London). His articles have appeared in *The Medical Observer*, *Australian Dr Weekly*, *Australian Psychologist*, *The Journal of Pediatrics and Child Health*, *The Journal of Psychohistory* and many other publications. His science and medical education writings have been recognised around the world, including by the American Medical Association. A lively and popular speaker, Dr Juan appears regularly on news and current affairs TV and radio programmes, covering any and all topics to do with being human in the world in which we live.

Born in California, Dr Juan was trained at the University of California at Berkeley. For 32 years, he taught in the Faculty of Education & Social Work at the University of Sydney, where he mentored many students while being affectionately known as "Dr Stevie". He retired in 2009 but remains the Ashley Montagu Fellow for the Public Understanding of Human Sciences.

Dr Stephen Juan welcomes questions and comments from readers and may be contacted at drstephenjuan@exemail.com.au OR

Dr Stephen Juan
c/o HarperCollins Publishers
13th Floor
201 Elizabeth Street
SYDNEY NSW 2000
AUSTRALIA

www.ingramcontent.com/pod-product-compliance
Lightning Source LLC
Chambersburg PA
CBHW022132020426
42334CB00015B/853